Surviving Your Medical Crisis

SURVIVING YOUR MEDICAL CRISIS

Strategies for finding the best doctors and hospitals for your care.

JERI GARNER, RN

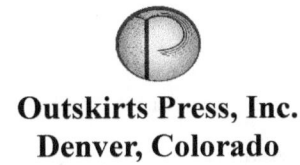

Outskirts Press, Inc.
Denver, Colorado

The opinions expressed in this manuscript are solely the opinions of the author and do not represent the opinions or thoughts of the publisher. The author has represented and warranted full ownership and/or legal right to publish all the materials in this book.

Surviving Your Medical Crisis
Strategies for finding the best doctors and hospitals for your care.
All Rights Reserved.
Copyright © 2009 Jeri Garner, RN
v2.0

Cover Photo © 2009 JupiterImages Corporation. All rights reserved - used with permission.

This book may not be reproduced, transmitted, or stored in whole or in part by any means, including graphic, electronic, or mechanical without the express written consent of the publisher except in the case of brief quotations embodied in critical articles and reviews.

Outskirts Press, Inc.
http://www.outskirtspress.com

ISBN: 978-1-4327-4510-3

Outskirts Press and the "OP" logo are trademarks belonging to Outskirts Press, Inc.

PRINTED IN THE UNITED STATES OF AMERICA

Disclaimer

This book has been written to help advise patients on ways to develop their personal medical plan. Everyone is unique, and this book does not presume to replace the need to communicate and work with a competent personal physician, and is not intended to replace professional medical care.

This book is dedicated to my husband John,
who is the love of my life.

And

To my Mother and Sister for their
courageous battle against cancer.

Contents

Introduction vii
Chapter 1 Finding The Best Hospitals For Your Care 1
Chapter 2 How to Find the Best Physicians for Your Care 39
Chapter 3 Understanding Your Disease Could Save Your Life ... 55
Chapter 4 Hospital Infectious Diseases 113
Chapter 5 Transfusions 165
Chapter 6 The ICU and Your Medical Plan 173
Chapter 7 Preventative Treatments 183
Chapter 8 Emergency Room Strategies 189
Conclusion 199
Medical Plan Summary 203
Terms to Know 207

Introduction

The sky was dark, with the exceptional flash of lightening, as the rain poured on your windshield. Just over the crest of the hill came another car headed right into your lane, your quick reaction sent your car off the road and tumbling end for end. As it came to a stop, you fade in and out of consciousness. Blood runs from your head and your leg and arm are pinned in the wreckage of the car. A Good Samaritan has called 911 and the Emergency Medical Service ambulance is on its way. As you are rushed from the accident scene, you are unaware that surviving the severe car accident may have been the easiest task of your day.

No one plans on needing emergency services or even on getting sick, but for most people, they will require medical attention at some point in their life. As we enter into the 21st century, the futuristic Star Trek medical techniques of long ago, are appearing to become more of a reality each and every day. Technology is changing at lightening speeds, and is moving just as fast in the healthcare setting. Can the hospitals and healthcare providers keep up? Although millions of patients are treated successfully every year, there are many that will not survive their hospital visit. You need to make sure that you have the ultimate support team in place that will give you every advantage to survive your medical crisis.

Where should you go? Who should you see? What treatments should be provided? Who will be your support system during your medical crisis? These are questions that are often not answered until we are faced with our own real crisis. Healthcare today presents a very complex scenario for even the most experience individual, let alone someone that is dealing with a medical crisis for the first time. It is time that we take charge of our health and our care, by developing a strong support system, before we are in the middle of a crisis.

My sister is a very well educated individual who has taken a very proactive stance with her health. Our mother had breast cancer 25 years ago, so my sister has been very faithful in her yearly health exams. She visited her doctor a year and a half ago, because she was experiencing pain in her breast and thought she felt a lump. The physician performed a mammogram and said that it was nothing to worry about, probably just a cyst and sent her on her way.

With the marriage of her daughter this past summer, and all the activities associated with that, she had put off her annual exam for a few months. She had planned on scheduling her appointment after the wedding, but before she could schedule it, she developed a pain in her neck. She went to her primary care physician, who ordered an X-ray of her neck.

The radiologist was pretty quick to say that it looked like a Hemangioma, which is a benign tumor, but he could not say for sure. She was then sent to a Neurologist who ordered a Magnetic Resonance Imaging (MRI) and a Bone Scan. The Neurologist looked at the MRI and said that the lesion in her neck was not a Hemangioma, but he was not sure what it was, but there were abnormal "hot spots" on her bone scan.

"Dr. Neurologist" wanted to know when her last Mammogram had been done. He recommended that she follow up with a Mammogram and Ultra Sound of her breast. The Mammogram was inconclusive, so the Ultra Sound was performed, and also left speculation of a clear diagnosis. A MRI was then performed, which indicated a mass in her breast. She was now referred to a surgeon, who finally performed a biopsy, which confirmed that she has breast cancer. She was then referred to an Oncologist for treatment options.

Her cancer had been undiagnosed (or misdiagnosed) a year and a half ago, and now, she has a confirmed diagnosis of cancer that looks like it has metastasized to her bones. When faced with facts like this, we tend to look at our health in a little different perspective. How could it have been missed a year and a half ago? Because of the size of the tumor at diagnosis, it should have been detected back then. Why did she get a different diagnosis every time she went to a different physician? She had questions, and she wanted answers.

Many patients have questions just like my sister did, but many do not have someone in the medical profession that they can turn to. My sister brought her questions to me and knew that I would provide her unbiased information about her condition. She also knew that I had her best interest in mind. Since she lives out of state, we spent hours on the phone, discussing her questions about tests, procedures, along with conventional and holistic treatment options. I became more than her sister, I became her support system.

We all need a support system that we can trust to have our best interest in mind. Those that really care about you are going to take the time to explain what is going on and put it into medical terms you can understand. The faith and trust you have in your healthcare team can often be shaken when test results generate conflicting results, and you may suddenly find yourself questioning everything that is happening to you. In order to make sure you have the best support team, you need the inside scoop. This book provides a very easy reference for evaluating hospitals and physicians. It also will offer information for the conditions that could require hospital attention, along with some standards of care for those diseases or conditions. It can help you evaluate the care you are being provided, and give you information on what treatments, and outcomes you could expect for your condition.

The risks associated with staying at, or even visiting the hospital, is not openly discussed in those television commercials the hospitals often produce. Not many people would want to go visit the hospital if their logo was….."GET YOUR FREE GERMS HERE", but in reality, the hospital can expose you to more deadly bacteria, than any other place that you visit. Sometimes we really do not want to know what "lies beneath", but with denial also comes the risk for not knowing the truth. The truth is not a bad thing and the truth can set us free. The fact is, we all face risks everyday, but what we do to reduce our risks, can save our lives. We take a chance every time we get in our car or cross the street, but we have learned from experience that things we do can reduce our risk for injury. The same is true for our health care, but it is often left to the consumer to find out how to reduce their chances of "catching something" while in the hospital, or avoiding a physician that does not meet their standards.

We have "plans" for finances, retirement, vacations, schedules, business, lessons, buildings, and it is time we develop a Medical Care Plan. The "4 legged stool" principle is a great model to adopt when building a strong medical team:

1. You need to have the right hospital for your condition.
2. You need the right physicians and healthcare workers.
3. You need to surround yourself with those that have your best interest in mind.
4. You need to be an active part of your medical team.

Without one of these basic principles, your health could be at risk, so build a strong Medical Portfolio before your medical crisis occurs and you will be armed with the necessary tools required for Surviving Your Medical Crisis.

CHAPTER 1

Finding The Best Hospitals For Your Care

Building your ultimate medical support team requires an understanding of how the medical community operates and where to find the best providers for your condition. A hospital is more than just a nice looking building or what flowers they have planted in their landscape. You need to know what goes on inside the hospital walls if you want accurate information.

As a registered nurse, I see first hand what goes on in a hospital setting, from a healthcare provider's perspective. It is like being in a family business, where you know your sibling's strengths and weaknesses. We understand that sometimes the family looks a little "dysfunctional", but it is what we do with that information that can make, or break the family unit. In order for the business to succeed, we need to have the most qualified people, doing the right thing, at the right time.

The same concept also applies to a "hospital family". Everyone at the hospital has their own strengths and weaknesses, from the physicians right on down to the lab techs. The imperfections can be magnified, and can have devastating consequences, when things are not done properly in a hospital setting. My clinical experiences with physicians, nurses, patients, administrations, executives and all other healthcare professionals, has provided me with a vast knowledge of how hospitals and healthcare providers function. You need to know who they are and how they operate before you entrust your life to them.

It became evident to me that patients do not always know what hospital they should go to for medical treatment, as I sat and watched a television commercial for one of the local hospitals. Hospitals are using the media to persuade people to come to their facility for their medical needs, but what is being portrayed in those commercials, may not be the "whole truth". In this very competitive healthcare market, you need to know more about your local hospitals than what they "want you to know". You need to know inside information about the hospital and if it could be an essential part of your healthcare team.

Does Size Matter?

One of the first areas to consider when making your hospital selection is the size, including how many beds they are licensed for. After working at different facilities in our metropolitan area, it did not take me long to see how different hospitals function and the wide range of services they offer. The small community hospitals often struggle just to get the basics done, while the mega hospitals can lose that personal touch. At the small hospital you are not just "the patient in room 1039B with COPD", you might actually have a name! If you are a patient at a large facility, you may be that patient in 1039B, but could also be offered new treatments that are not available at the small facility. Understanding what is important to you can help direct your choice of hospitals and physicians. No matter how big or small a hospital is, it needs to put customer service at the forefront.

It is often the little things that a hospital does or does not do that can send big messages to patients and their family members. I had someone stop by one hospital to drop something off for me one day. He said that the greeter at the front desk was less than competent.

She did not know how to locate me, even with all the information he provided, and then on top of that, she was rude. This should have been a very easy task for the receptionist to master, but all it did was make a terrible impression on the visitor. I have traveled to several different hospitals that have required me to "meet" the hospital receptionist and I can attest that many hospitals have figured out that their customer service starts at the front door, but it also travels throughout the hallways, elevators and the cafeteria.

I once knew a patient that "visited" a hospital she was considering for her elective surgery, just to have lunch. As she sat in the cafeteria, she was able to listen to the staff's conversations, and gained a wealth of information about the hospital. The hospitals do stress patient confidentiality, and it was not that she heard patient names, but she heard about the hospital drama. She collected an amazing amount of information over the two hours she spent in the cafeteria. She left with more than she ever bargained for, and decided to schedule the surgery at a different hospital.

Do not get me wrong, there are a lot of hospitals out there that are getting the job done, but no one is perfect. As any health care worker will tell you, they have the insight to know what goes on at the hospital, which physicians you want to go to, and units you want to avoid. Nurses would often say in our clinical groups, that a certain hospital is on my "never take me there" list. During a nursing school clinical rotation, I watched in horror as a physician dropped an instrument on the floor and then picked it up and put it into the comatose patient. As a student, I lacked the confidence to question the doctor's practices, but today, that is not a problem. Deciding which hospital you will go to may be based on preference, but I say a little knowledge goes a long way. As healthcare providers we see things from a different perspective, but most patients do not have our privileged medical perspective.

Most of the time patients arrive at the hospital in an emergency situation, without much planning or forethought. They see a doctor that they do not know and are provided a diagnosis in a language they may not understand. We have a patient, with a new diagnosis, in a new place, with terms that they do not understand, but they are suppose to trust those strangers with their life. Do you see a problem with this picture?

In the emergency situations, patients and family members just want someone to "make them better". Sometimes the family members are present to hear the report, and other times they are not. Studies have reported that the patient may only retain fifty percent of what the physician tells them after hearing key words like "cancer", so now we are faced not only with the lack of understanding, but also the lack of knowledge due to the low information retention. Add in the fact that many doctors and nurses are overworked and understaffed, and the patient is the one that suffers the most. What a place to be.

What happens in these situations can put you or your loved ones at risk. I have always said that you need to be your own "patient advocate", and in order for this to be done effectively, you and your loved ones need to have information about your condition, your doctors, nurses, hospital, treatments and the risks involved. In order to make informed decisions about a hospital, you need to understand a little more about what services they have available for your healthcare needs.

The Services

Hospitals come in many shapes and sizes. They differ in the medical equipment they own and the treatments they can provide. Hospitals are in competition with other local hospitals and most have marketing departments that strategize over how they are going to get your business.

They take surveys of the community to see if people recognize the hospital's name or if they would visit their facility when they get sick. With the fierce competition, some hospitals have even brought in former hotel CEOs to manage the facility. The philosophy of "if you build it, they will come", has changed the focus of the healthcare industry. The local community hospitals often struggle as people are willing to travel quite a distance for medical treatment. All it takes is for you or someone you love to have a "bad" experience at one hospital for you to drive miles to get to a different one the next time.

Because the states do not want hospitals popping up all over, they have applied what is called a "Certificate of Need". Anyone wanting to start a hospital or add onto an existing one must show that there is a need for it in the community, and likewise for technology or certain diagnostic equipment. For this reason, not all hospitals have certain equipment, like MRI machines. If you have ever been to a hospital that needs to transport you via an ambulance to get your necessary MRI, you understand how important it is to have the diagnostic equipment on the hospital premises. It is important to ask what diagnostic equipment is on the premises and when it is staffed. Many small hospitals do not staff the MRI or CT with radiologist on the weekends, so your test could be delayed, even if they do have the equipment.

My husband, John was experiencing abdominal pain one Easter weekend and needed to go to the hospital. I was out of town at the time, so our son took him to a local facility. I called frequently for updates, but could only get bits and pieces of information. He felt it would just require a quick trip to the ER, but they ended up admitted him, for "tests". I called the next day and he told me that they were keeping him another day. By this point I wanted to know what was going on, and felt that there was something that John was not telling me, because I was out of town. As it turned out, the only problem he really had was that it was a holiday weekend, and the test would not be "available" until Monday.

The hospital did not want the liability of sending him home without the test, but really did not want to tell him he would have to wait 2 days before the test would be done. This type of scenario costs you time, money and increases your risk for exposure to deadly diseases.

So do you choose a small hospital or a large one? Do you want one with all the "bells and whistles", or do you want one close to home? Large facilities may offer state-of-the-art equipment for diagnostics and surgical procedures. These are also the hospitals that usually are "teaching" facilities, which means they have ties to a medical school, with residents practicing at their hospital. The focus at these hospitals tends to be more on research and the newest techniques or treatments. The size of a hospital can matter, but you must look at each individual facility separately to gain an accurate view of what goes on inside the hospital walls.

Doctors and Residents and Interns, Oh My!

Because of the research often being conducted at larger hospitals, we may find top notch physicians that specialize in the area being researched. The residents may also be gaining valuable experience under physicians that are pioneering the way in medical research. We will cover some of this in more detail under the *Selecting a Physician* chapter.

You must ask yourself if you like having medical students, interns and residents "drooling" over your case, or if you just like your primary care attending to your care, as it would be at the small community hospital. The larger hospitals tend to have the necessary staff at the hospital 24/7. I have worked at both types of hospitals and can see benefits to both situations. At the teaching hospital, there were so many times that something would go wrong with a patient in the middle of the night, and the residents would come running. It was nice to have someone right there to assist in the direct care, as apposed to paging the doctor, then waiting for the return call. Physicians must trust their residents with their patients, but the residents are only rounding with a particular physician for a period of time.

Make Sure the Hospital is Accredited

You may have several hospitals to choose from, but no matter what one you select, make sure that they are approved by the Joint Commission on Accreditation of Healthcare Organizations (JCAHO) or by the American Osteopathic Association (AOA) which are a Healthcare Facilities Accreditation Program (HFAP). These organizations make regular visits to hospitals for physical inspections of the facilities along with evaluations of the hospital's procedures and policies.

Results of the JCAHO surveys can be found at http://www.qualitycheck.org/consumer/searchQCR.aspx. For a listing of Osteopathic hospitals approved by AOA can be viewed at: http://www.osteopathic.org.

Search for a hospital by organization name, zip code or state, but once you select the hospital, click on "View Accreditation Quality Report" for detailed information. The report will show you how the hospital compares to other hospitals in your state, as well as nationwide. If the hospital has received any awards for their specialized services, they will also be listed, along with the year of the award. The JCAHO or AOA audit is a very important part of the hospital and much planning and implementation goes into preparation for the surveys.

CMS Hospital Reports

The Center for Medicare and Medicaid (CMS) also collects information from the hospitals that everyone should know about. It is not an inclusive list of everything that goes on at a hospital but it provides a good place to start. The CMS has provided a website to compare hospitals in your community and across the nation by logging online to: http://www.hospitalcompare.hhs.gov.

This site allows you to look at what they call "core measures" for each hospital. Some of the information generated by CMS reports can also be found on the JCAHO site. The hospitals that are striving for improved scores can provide you with the confidence that they are capable of taking care of you in your time of need. The collection of information is abstracted on a random selection basis through independent reporting services. Medical charts are randomly selected for the auditing process. Because of this randomization, there is always the chance that some "good" things go unnoticed, or that the "bad" things do not get reported.

There are a limited number of categories that data is currently collected from and almost all of it relates to adult patients. There are new categories being added all the time so check back frequently. The information provided can be over a year old, but if you want to make comparisons and see where your favorite hospital ranks next to national averages, or their local competitors, then you have come to the right place. These reports can offer so much information, that you might be a little overwhelmed, so let us try to break it down, for easy digestion.

Medicare Data Categories

The categories provided on the website are broken down into certain conditions or procedures as listed below:

1. Medical Conditions: Hearth attack, heart failure, chronic lung disease, pneumonia, diabetes in adults, chest pain.

2. Surgical Procedures:

- **a. Cardiac:** Heart and blood vessels, angioplasty procedures, heart bypass surgery, heart valve operations, insertion of heart defibrillators, pacemaker implants, major heart and blood vessel procedures, head and neck blood vessel operations.
- **b. Abdominal:** Gallbladder removal, hernia operations, intestine operations, stomach and esophagus operations, neck, back and extremities.
- **c. Neck, Back and Extremities** (Arms and Legs) : Back fusion, neck fusion, back and neck operations, upper and lower extremity operations, bone procedures, bone removal.
- **d. Bladder, Kidney and Prostate**: Kidney and bladder operations, other kidney and bladder operations, prostate removal.
- **e. Female Reproductive:** Female reproductive operations.

Report Comparisons

This website provides general information about the hospital and the outcomes related to the various areas of care. Under the General Information we can see if the facility provides emergency services, how often the best plan of care for a particular condition is provided, results of their care for certain conditions and what pervious patients have said about the facility. In short, there are those that have studied certain conditions, and based on those outcomes, have made recommendations for how other patients with those conditions should be cared for. Not everyone fits into a box, but there are certain methods of care that have been "proven" to be beneficial to the patient with certain types of conditions or diseases.

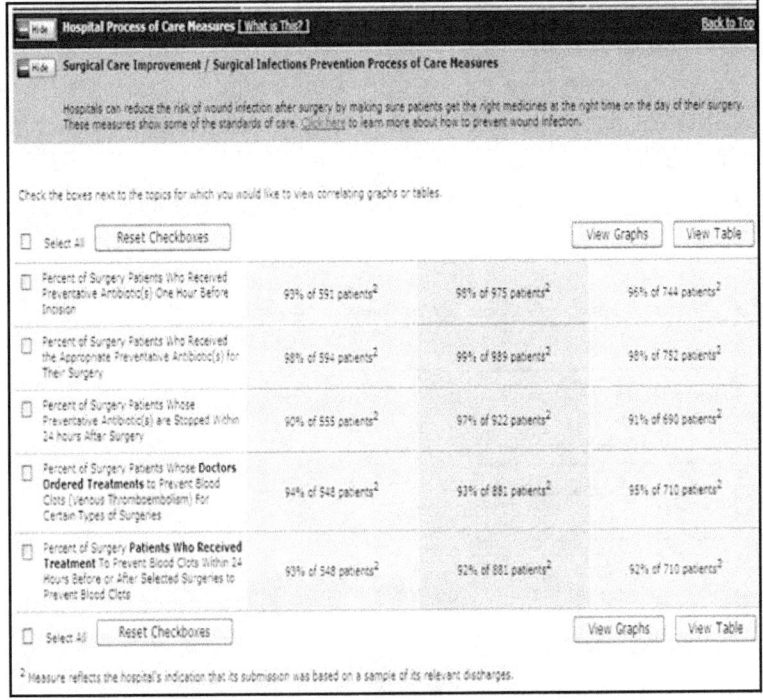

(graph 1 used by permission of CMS)

Graph 1 provides a sample report of data collected from three hospitals from the CMS survey. We can also see how many cases the hospital has treated compared to other facilities in the area. It stands to reason, if the facility is not reporting because they do not have the minimum number of cases required to report, we might want to go somewhere else for that type of treatment.

It comes down to one simple question: Would you rather go to a hospital that takes care of thousands of patients with your type of

◄ SURVIVING YOUR MEDICAL CRISIS

condition every year, or just a few? In the medical field we can have very intelligent people, with a lot of degrees after their name, but it is experience that takes them from being a novice to an expert. We need to make informed decision about our healthcare, and often that begins by doing some research.

Elective Surgery Reports

CMS collects data on elective surgery, where we can compare not only local hospitals, but national averages. This information may be a little hard to decipher, but should provide a general idea of how effective the hospital is managing their surgical patients. In *graph 2*, we can see that the national average for patients to receive preventative antibiotics within one hour of surgical incision is 84%, the average for Michigan hospitals is 89%, and all three of the hospitals selected are above that average for this question.

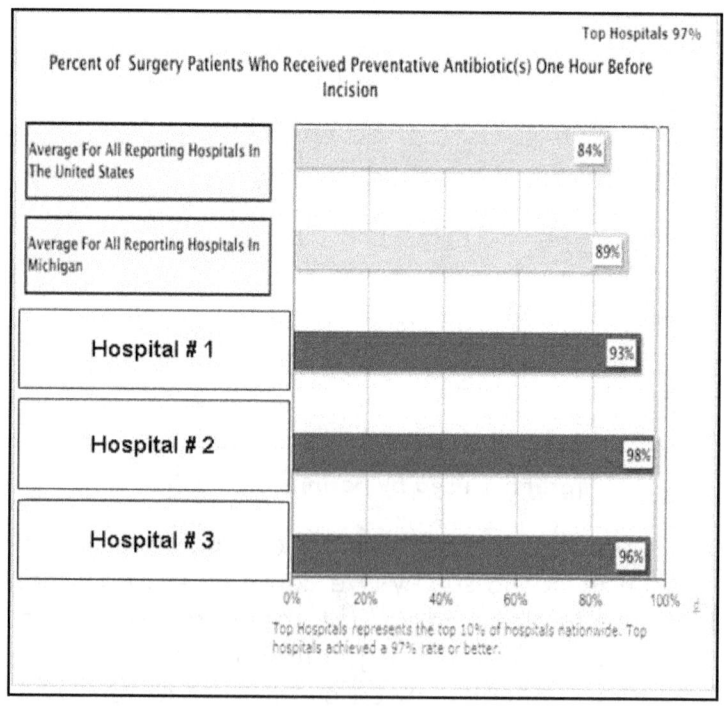

(graph 2 used by permission of CMS)

FINDING THE BEST HOSPITALS FOR YOUR CARE

Therapeutic Treatments

In *graph 3* we can see the variance of heart attack treatments provided by each of the selected hospitals. The first facility does not take care of very many patients with this condition, and we want a hospital that has experience. The second facility listed is "perfect" at providing an ACE inhibitor medication for their heart attack patients. Wow, we should like the sounds of "perfection" when it comes to our healthcare provider. The last one is right in between the national average and the state average. The chances of receiving the care that we need at this hospital are very good.

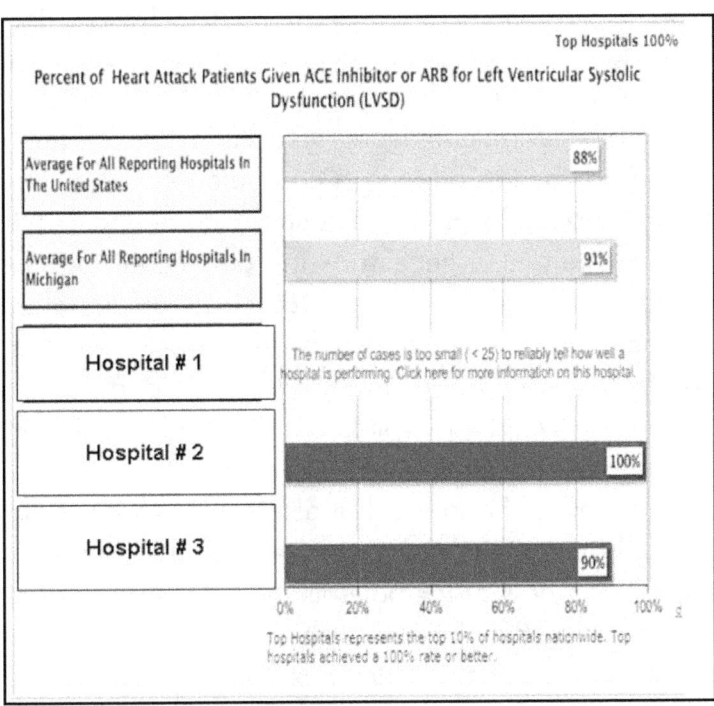

(graph 3 used by permission of CMS)

Centers of Excellence

Hospitals often receive national recognition for their services and specialties they provide. The hospitals have to pass a stringent regiment before they will be given these titles and they are usually honored to say they have received this type of recognition. Even though hospitals may take a different approach for treating certain conditions, those facilities awarded "Center of Excellence" are 50 percent more likely to have physicians and nurses that have specialized training in that specific area of medicine. In general it means that the patient's complication rate may be lower and the hospital stay could be shorter.

Patients that receive treatment at a Center of Excellence are more likely to be provided comprehensive follow-up care after they leave the hospital. Understand that just because a hospital is a "Center of Excellence" for one specialty, it may not be for others, so be specific when inquiring about the Excellence awards. Some hospitals offer specialized services, but the treatment may still be limited.

For example, "Maple Hospital" specializes in treating stroke patients, and has begun offering a computerized assessment via a webcam, of the patients at "Oak Hospital". If an intervention such as removal of the clot is necessary, the patient will be transferred out to "Maple Hospital" because "Oak Hospital" is not equipped to handle that type of intervention. If you live between "Maple and Oak Hospitals", it could save you time, money and your life if you went directly to "Maple Hospital" if you had stroke symptoms. When making your hospital selection, you should consider what the hospital is capable of handling, but also some other criteria.

Not only should you be aware of the "Centers of Excellence" for each hospital, but how many patients they see on those units every year, and how long they have met the criteria for this recognition. A hospital that has been a Center of Excellence for 5 years has met the standards of care for a longer period of time than one that received the award 6 months ago. In a Center of Excellence hospital, the routines and processes that have been proven to be effective in patient care have had the chance to become second nature for many of the healthcare providers at a hospital with 5 years of recognition.

Patient Responses

Previous patient's responses can provide us with a well rounded assessment of the hospital. Anyone that has been in a "service" type of occupation will tell you when people are NOT happy with the services they receive, they will tell 10 other people on average. After working in the hospital, I will be the first to tell you that there are some people that you could never make "happy". In this survey, you take the good with the bad and hope that the scores are pretty accurate. Graph 4 contains an example of an evaluation for how well the physicians and nurses were able to; communicate, control pain, explain medications, provide detailed discharge instructions, rate the cleanliness of the rooms, the hospital rating, and if they would recommend the hospital. If the national average was 70 percent for cleanliness of the rooms, you might wonder what was going on with a facility that only scored 54 percent. Although this may sound trivial, proper sanitation of the rooms could help reduce your risk of acquiring hospital-bacteria.

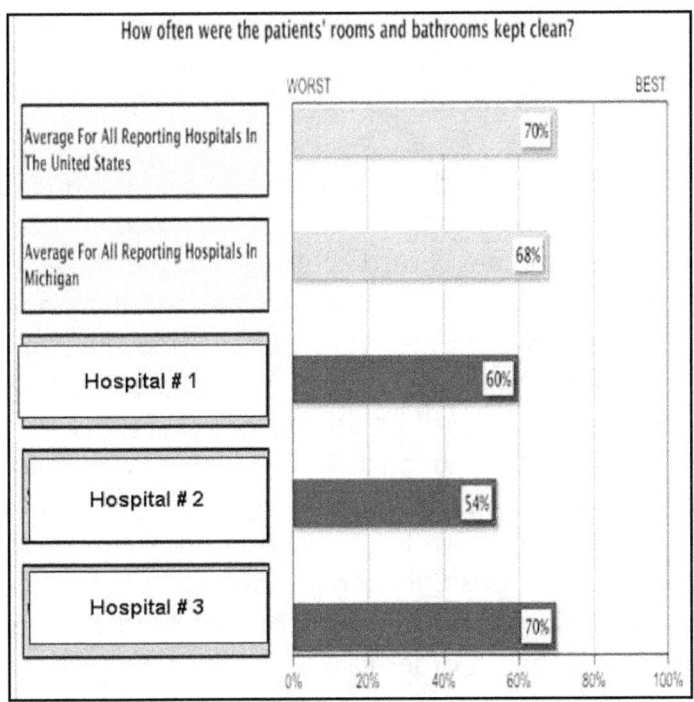

(Graph 4 used by permission of CMS)

Comparison of the different websites will give an inside look at how the patients are treated, the hospital infection rates and what other patients have discovered.

Key factors to remember when performing hospital comparisons on the CMS website:

1. **The Hospital Process of Care** section is how well the hospital cared for their patients. Percentages and number of cases in this category are more of a factor as we want a hospital with experience.
2. **The Outcomes** section provides mortality rates. This is good information to know, because if one hospital has a high mortality rate; we might want to avoid making this our hospital of choice. Remember, no hospital is perfect and many factors can contribute to a patient's mortality.
3. **The Patient Survey** gives us practical information on the caregivers and the hospital in general. Sometimes the best advice comes from those that have been there.

Medicare is always adding to the data they are requesting from the hospitals, so check frequently to see the updated information. There are other websites that are also starting to collect hospital data, which will just make the access to this information more readily available, but always consider the source. Some sites are focused on patient comments which can be insightful, but should not be what we exclusively base our decisions on.

Take the CMS information and combine it with some of the other sites to make sure you are getting the whole picture. Some information that is collected is generated by patient responses to a survey after a hospital visit. If hospitals are striving to improve their quality of care, they need to know where they stand… the good, the bad and the ugly, but in order for them to know that, you must fill out the surveys if you receive one.

Quality of care should be top on the priority list for all hospitals, but just as with any other business, especially in this current economy, there is always the money factor. Even though the hospital may be portrayed as the "wellness center", designed to serve the public, they are still operating as a business. Medicine is big business and it is the financial aspect that keeps them functioning. Most hospitals will provide you with their financial statement, and it can be a very valuable tool in your research. If the hospital is making cuts in their budget, you may be the recipient of those adjustments. Make sure to check the date on the financial report, as it could be over a year old, and a lot can change in a short period of time.

It is important to look at the number of patients that the hospital is reporting on for the CMS data, and what kind of outcomes the patients have had. Some hospital reports may not reflect the total truth when it comes to statistics. Statistics may place a hospital high in the national rankings, but in reality, they do not have the facilities to handle the critical patients, so if the patient becomes critical, they are transferred out to a larger facility. The larger facility is now the one that will hold the patient's records for reporting measures. If the patient dies, the large facility will hold the "death record", while the smaller hospital looks like it did not have any patients with complications. It is a tricky system when it comes to reporting, and things may not be accurately portrayed in the statistics.

Hospital Considerations

There are pros and cons for both the large and small hospitals, so evaluate what is important to you. Research the online sites provided in this chapter to aid in your investigation and talk to your family and friends about the care they have received from these hospitals. Go visit the hospital and see first hand what goes on, and what the staff is saying or doing. Check out the food, the cleanliness and competency of the staff. Remember that a picture is worth a thousand words.

You can have things go wrong at any hospital but if you are an active part of your medical team, and you have a great support system in place, you can feel confident you will receive the level of care that your condition requires.

The website: http://www.hospital-data.com/ provides general information about hospitals across the United States, such as the size, how many nurses and physicians the hospital has on staff, their accreditations, and much more. This could be an easy way for you to collect relative information pertaining to your hospital search. When selecting a hospital, you do not want to pick the one that you think you can "live with"; you want to pick the one that you cannot "live without". If you would like assistance in this process, you can go to www.MyMedicalAdvisor.net as they offer a consulting service for developing your medical plan.

Insurance or Not?

When selecting a hospital we will need to consider how we are going to pay for their services. It does not matter if the hospital visit is as an outpatient or inpatient, the insurance or the patient will be billed for the services rendered. Insurance or lack thereof can play a big part in your care. Understanding how the hospital gets paid may provide some insight for cutting through the hospital bureaucracy.

Medicare generally sets the "standards" for payment on services rendered, as they tell the hospital how much they will pay for certain services. For example, if a patient comes to the hospital for a mastectomy, Medicare has approved a flat rate for the entire hospital stay, no matter if it is for 1 day or 3 days. The average length of stay (LOS) may be 1.5 days for this procedure. If the hospital bill is $20,000 and they can discharge the patient within 1 day, the hospital makes more money as they can fill "the bed" with another patient that much sooner. It may also cut down on the number of staff required to take care of the patients, and in turn, provides cost saving measures to the hospital.

I would like to tell you that money does not play a factor in treatment decisions, but the bottom line is, money plays a very big role in the hospital setting. It does not matter if you are AIG, one of the automotive companies, or a hospital, if you want to stay in

FINDING THE BEST HOSPITALS FOR YOUR CARE

business, you need to generate revenue. Some CFO's are great managers and have made great financial decisions for the hospital, but the patient is not always the top priority.

No Insurance

There are 46 million Americans without healthcare and that number is growing every day. Often the uninsured are charged as much as three times what a patient with insurance is charged. If you must make a visit to a hospital, and you do not have insurance, understand that hospitals are required to provide emergency care to stabilize the patient whether they have insurance or not.

There are different rules for non-profit and for-profit hospitals. You need to check with your local hospitals to see what their policies are for treating those without insurance, if this applies to you. There may be some hospitals in your area that provide care to individuals without insurance. If you received care from a hospital, and you do not have insurance, you need to contact the hospital's billing department to see what can be done for your situation.

I knew a lady that was visiting from another country and ended up delivering her pre-mature baby while in Michigan. Needless to say, she had no insurance, and the bill for her, and the baby in intensive care for weeks was almost a million dollars. The hospital had a fund for such cases, and the entire bill was written off.

My friend (who was a citizen of the United States) went to this same hospital with her son for outpatient surgery. They only had catastrophic insurance and the bill was $3000, so she had to make monthly payments for the entire amount. When her checks were not as much as the hospital wanted, they harassed her and threaten to take her to court. You need to know the right people to talk to when negotiating your bill, so start by speaking with the financial department of the hospital. Do not be intimated, just tell them your situation, and see what they can do for you. Sometimes the total debt can be significantly reduced, so let them know what you can pay on the bill each month. Many people are forced into bankruptcy over medical bills, and if that occurs, then the hospital stands to get nothing. Let them know that you are willing to work with them. Most hospitals would rather get $100 a month over the next 30 months, than not to get paid at all.

No matter if you have insurance or not, you need to check the hospital bill for errors. You can obtain a detailed list for services rendered from the hospital and then "go to work". Make sure the dates, diagnosis, medications provided, etc. are all correct. Remember that any errors you find is money back in your pocket. Some insurance companies will even give you a "bonus" for errors you find on the bill that results in them not paying for erroneous charges. I have also find hospital documentation even with the wrong name listed on the patient account, so check everything.

If You Have Insurance

If you have insurance you will want to know if your local hospitals participate with your insurance, which is called a preferred provider. This may help you decide which hospital to go to if you have a choice. Hospitals will often offer discounts for insurances that they participate with and that should affect how much you pay for their services. Do not feel that you are limited to only the hospitals or physicians that participate with your insurance, just understand that services from non-provider hospitals may require you to pay the entire bill. Contact your insurance company for details on your coverage plan and make sure you read the fine print.

Co-pays and deductibles are also factors in your total bill. My first baby was delivered by a caesarean section, which required an anesthesiologist service. The anesthesiologist group did not participate with my insurance, so I was responsible for the entire bill. There are times that physician or hospitals will accept the amount the insurance pays as the total payment, but this does not happen very often. Make sure before you have a procedure that your insurance is going to pay for it.

Approval is required a head of time for some services, so make sure you ask a head of time how much a procedure will cost and if your insurance will cover it. It might even be necessary for you to call your insurance company for verification. The way treatments or procedures get billed can also play a part in the insurance payment.

My husband John had injured his foot, and the physician offered either physical therapy or surgery as treatment options. We opted for the therapy as it sounded like a better alternative to surgery. After several weeks of therapy, we got our first bill from the physical therapy company. The insurance company did not cover any of the invoice. When I contacted the insurance company, they said that the diagnosis did not meet their "requirement for treatment", yet if he had decided to have surgery, it would have been covered.

After working with the physician, we found something had been coded wrong, so we were able to resubmit the claim to the insurance and all we ended up paying was our deductable. Things often get coded wrong, and it is common place to see services get rejected. Just because you get an invoice for services rendered, make sure that it has been sent to the insurance company first. If you ever get a claim denied for payment, contact the provider and find out what codes were used on the claim. You will also need to contact your insurance company and ask why it was denied. I have had several claims denied (for whatever reason), and by becoming a mediator between the facility and the insurance company, I have been able to get the insurance company to pay the claims. You must understand how many people are associated with just one claim, and like anything else, there is the chance for error or misinterpretation of the information received.

Additional Expenses-

You also need to be aware that you may receive additional bills from services outside of the hospital. In order to reduce financial obligations, many hospitals have out-sourced services for their facility. One hospital that I worked for outsourced the anesthesiologist, emergency room physicians, radiologist, pharmacist, dieticians, information technology group and physical therapy (just to name a few). Just because you had the surgery at the hospital, if you received services from any of these departments, you may receive an additional bill.

When I had my first baby; I received a bill from a doctor that I did not know. Because my baby was 11 pounds, he was seen by a specialist unbeknownst to me. It was a standard protocol at that hospital for any of the babies over 10 pounds to be assessed for causation of their size. My husband is 6'9" and weighed 11 pounds 6 ounces when he was born, so I probably could have told them why he was so big. Even though it was a genetic thing, I still got the bill! The policies probably had my best interest in mind, but you just need to be aware of these possible charges.

Telephone and television service are common services that may require you to pay extra. Most hospitals allow you to use your cell phone inside the building, but you may want to find out what the hospital's policy is on cell phone use. Some hospitals may still want to make money from the service fee they charge for a room phone.

Due to many cost cutting measures, some hospitals are asking that you bring in your own toiletries. If you have a planned visit, you might want to take your own "supplies", but remember that the hospital is a "sick" place, so try to take things that you can throw away when you get ready to leave. Most hospitals still have some supplies on site for those patients that do not have access to their own from home, but you may have to ask for them.

Wireless Internet is also a new feature for many hospitals so inquiring about this service and associated fees could help you decide if you are going to bring your laptop to the hospital. Some hospitals are now offering a room with a public computer access. Anyone visiting or a patient is allowed to use these computers, but with that also may come exposure to contagious diseases. Just make sure that you wash your hands after using one of the hospital's supplied computers, and keep all cuts and scraps covered with a bandage to avoid contamination.

FINDING THE BEST HOSPITALS FOR YOUR CARE

Even though the hospital will provide your necessary medications, you can ask your physician if you can take your own from home, especially if you do not have insurance. Sometimes you can get several bottles for the cost of one pill at the hospital. Your own medications can provide great savings, but **NEVER** take any medications without your doctor's permission, as this could put your own life at risk. The nurse should know about any medications that you have in your possession, and if they have not been approved by the hospital staff for administration, they need to be sent home. There is enough risk at the hospital without you creating any more.

The Hospital Bill
1. Check to see if the hospital accepts your insurance.
2. Read the fine print on your insurance policy and understand the terms.
3. Find out if the hospital treats uninsured patients.
4. If you do not have insurance, communicate with the hospital and see what type of payment plan can be negotiated.
5. Just because the hospital participates with your insurance, make sure that all of the ancillary services do as well.
6. Check your bill for errors, and notify your insurance company if you find any.
7. Notify the hospital of the errors and request an updated statement from them.
8. Obtain clearance on medical procedures before treatment is completed.
9. Ask if you can take your own medication.
10. Never take any medications (including over the counter) while in the hospital unless your healthcare providers have approved.
11. Ask what other services (i.e., phone, TV) that the hospital offers that will require upfront payment.
12. Inquire if cell phone usage is permitted in the hospital.

Electronic Health Records

The electronic health record (EMR) has come to the fore front for many hospitals and can play a very important part in your hospital visit. I truly believe that the EMR has a place in the hospital as it can provide fast, efficient information to the healthcare staff, while providing allergy verifications to medications. With faster results, we should expect faster treatment and a sooner recovery. This does not guarantee that just because your hospital is "high tech" with computers on every corner that you are going to get better care. It just means that the potential is there.

With the possibility for improved care also comes the risk associated with this new technology. Physician, nurses, and the rest of the hospital staff are now faced with a total change in their process. Errors can occur when the wrong order gets placed or even when the order gets missed. For the patient, this means that life saving treatments might not be provided, or you might get the wrong treatment. The errors are usually generated when there is a break down in the interface between the clinical staff and the computer. JCAHO reports that harmful medication errors related to the EMR technology have occurred, and the numbers could rise, as more hospitals get on the technology train.

In 2006, JCAHO reported that 43,372 harmful medication events occurred as a direct result of computer utilization, out of 176,409 total medication errors. Every day errors occur that go unreported, so these numbers in actuality could be much higher than what is being reported. Insuring that the staff has adequate training is a first line of defense for error prevention. The effectiveness and safety of the computerized system ultimately depends on the clinicians using it. The varying degrees of computer literacy can pose a problem for general education classes for the new system. Some of the clinical staff is very computer savvy, while others do not even know what a mouse is. Some can type, while others do know even know where the letter "T" is on the keyboard.

Even though education is provided, scheduling physicians,

nurses, nursing assistants, unit clerks, nurse practitioners, physician assistants and the rest of the hospital staff for education classes can be a huge undertaking. There could be thousands that need to be trained, and many hospitals do not have the adequate staff for this necessary training.

Everyone is trying to take care of their patients, and it can be difficult to carve a few hours out of their day, to learn something new. Many practitioners do not receive adequate amounts of training, due to the time constraints, but each hospital is responsible for initiating mandatory education and evaluating their staff after training. To adequately learn the new computerized system, the practitioners need to have the ability to attend classes and then be provided "test patients" to practice on. For those that do attend education classes, the training material for each of these practitioners needs to be customized for easy application. This focused study can be beneficial when taking time out of a busy practitioner's day. General navigation of the entire EMR also needs to be provided so the clinicians know where to find the data they will need to take care of their patients.

The hospitals that have the most compliance also provide the staff with the online practice resources that allow them to sharpen their skills prior to utilizing the computerized system on the patients. Many hospitals provide this online resource to their physicians and nurses, but there are many that do not. The hospital needs to also put a high priority on education, training and continued 24/7 support for the computerized system. We put high standards on individuals that want to drive a car, and it is not just for their safety, but for those around them. The same principle applies to the integration of the computerized system into the hospital setting.

Safety of the patient needs to be the top priority when considering the EMR. When a hospital says that they are 70-80 percent ready for a "go-live", that is a little scary. This tells us that they know about the 20-30 percent of things that are "wrong" with the system, but it does not figure in the "unknown variables". In all reality, the hospital's system could be only 50 percent ready for "go-live". With those odds, it would be like saying you have a 50 percent chance of something going wrong with your care, which could even cost you your life. At this time, most errors are not generally computer generated, but there is a responsibility of the hospital to make sure safety measures are in place before they implement this technology. Hospitals need to aim for the 100 percent readiness prior to initiation of the EMR, because there will always be problems that are discovered after the "go-live" application is implemented.

Hospitals all over the nation have EMRs, but there are several computerized systems that they can choose from, or they might have an information technology team that has designed and created a program specifically designed for a hospital. No matter what modality the hospital has selected, the front-line informatics clinicians need to insure that the system will function well with other hospital computer programs. Clinicians with front-line experience should be key components in planning, testing and assessment of clinical process as it relates to system integration.

Since this is a new world for many clinicians, there is often a lack of IT experience by the clinicians, and vise versa for the IT department, who often lack clinical experience. It takes strong leadership and organization for these two worlds to mesh for a safe electronic system. Those that oversee the electronic system need to consider how this will affect the clinicians work flow along with the safety of the patient. Key elements can be missed if those in authority do not understand the functionality of the system.

A week after one hospital "go-live" the project manager went out on medical leave and I was asked to cover for her during this time. After a few days of getting things settled down, I told the team that I needed to go work the floor, and take care of patients. With this first hand experience, I was able to evaluate the work flow process for the computer application and the nursing process. Sometimes things look really good in the concept phase, but once you try and put it into action, you can see the flaws. I knew this computerized system inside and out, as I had played a key role in design, testing, training and implementation of the EMR. I probably could have worked the system in my sleep, but carrying a team of patients gave a whole new perspective.

I met with my IT team for lunch after taking care of 5 patients (which may be a low number in today's standards), and my practical evaluation told me that it was more than we had expected. We had taken things that looked really good in practice, but when combined with reality, we actually created a monster. We went back to the drawing board on several items and rethought the workflow process. We wanted our system to be functional but also user friendly. If the hospital wants a safe EMR application, those in leadership positions need to understand what the clinicians are going through, to truly understand the impact of the new technology on their practice. For the consumer, there needs to be the understanding of how this computerized method of record keeping can impact patient care and the risk associated with it.

The computer is a key part of patient care today, but as a patient, you want to know where the hospital is in their implementation process of the EMR. The first few weeks after a "go-live" can be pretty rough if testing of the system and education have not been implemented properly. Some facilities just "pull the paper" and all orders will be placed directly into the computer from that day forward. Others may take a single phase approach and have the system be rolled out in different segments. With either method, there are risks associated with the integration of the computer and patient care.

Multi-hospital facilities often have the advantage of initiating the system in one hospital, and then learning from their mistakes, so they will make the necessary changes, before they roll out the next hospital's system. Smaller hospitals do not have this luxury and may find themselves "reinventing the wheel". Understanding what EMR the hospital has in place, and any plans they have for future updates of the system, is something that you want to know prior to your admission. There are very few regulatory measures in place for hospital electronic systems at this time, so it is left to the consumer to ask the questions. Strategic planning, testing, accountability, training and education all need to be implemented if the hospital wants a safe EMR.

Your Physician and the EMR

If your physicians have been practicing for any length of time, they more than likely learned to write their orders on paper. Even though the writing was not always legible, the physician knew what he wrote. When all the orders are to be placed directly into the computer, someone has to do.

Some physicians are very computer savvy, and well, let's just say, others aren't. When training practitioners to work with the EMR, I could tell in the first 5 seconds how successful the training session was going to be. I would just ask the practitioner to "log in" which required their first initial, last name and their password. I knew if they struggled with that small task, that I had my work cut out for me. The success rate for getting those "computer challenged" physicians to actually use the computerized system was also drastically reduced. The hospital has just taken a very capable physician that has been practicing medicine for say, 25 years, and has totally changed their process. It would be equivalent to us cutting off a surgeon's arm and telling him he will now need to perform surgery with one hand. He would be able to do it if the desire is high enough and he has the time to learn the new techniques.

For most physicians, especially surgeons, time is money. The more surgeries they are able to perform in a day, the more money they will make. Some surgeons have gone to hiring Physician Assistants or Nurse Practitioners to assist with this change in their practice. If you are at a teaching hospital, then most of the residents put the orders in for the physicians they are following, and this situation can pose its own risks. The residents often represent the younger generation and are definitely more adapt to computers, but they are still learning the medical aspect of caring for patients.

It could take a good ten years of transition in this field, as we will have physicians that will be retiring, new physicians coming in to take their positions, and those in the middle that will be forced to jump on the electronic train call the EMR. Some facilities are still allowing the physician to write their orders, then, either the nurse, unit clerk or pharmacist enters the order into the computer. With this type of system, we are still back to "reading" the physician's hand writing. The more methods used to place orders also increases your risk for errors.

There is a high enough risk with the physician placed orders, let alone the physician writing them, and someone else transcribing them. In this design, there could be several "transcriptions" for just one order, and this is certainly not the most effective, or desirable method of order placement. The question of who is best suited for the order process still remains when you have clinicians that are not able to navigate a computer system. You need to know how orders are place at your hospital, and who places the orders as each hospital may be a little different. Because there are so many ways to implement and manage the way the electronic records are kept, there can also be different "flaws" at different facilities. The hospital is not the auto assembly line, where the same thing is done, minute by minute, hour by hour, by the same robots.

Orders are placed minute by minute, but by different people, in different ways, for different patients. I have found that if the computerized system "allows" people to place an order the "wrong way", someone will find that way, even though they have been taught how to correctly place the order. It is like going to McDonalds and ordering a cheeseburger without ketchup, and getting to the car and finding out you got chicken nuggets! It went in the computer, but somehow, it got messed up, and it is generally related to human error. You need to know how computer savvy your physician is, how orders are placed and who puts the orders into the computer, for your own safety.

Integrated Computerized Systems

Errors can be caused by clinical, clerical or technical reasons, so to limit the technical difficulties; the hospital IT department needs effective planning and understanding of clinical processes as it relates to the computerized system. Many departments in the hospitals such as the pharmacy or the laboratory may already have an electronic data system in place. The cost of an EMR is astronomical for most hospitals with millions of dollars budgeted for the major project, not including the amount it takes to maintain the system. Many hospitals are not changing the computerized systems that they already have in place, but are integrating the new computer application with their existing software programs. This integration may be like trying to make a Ford bumper fit your Mercedes Benz. It takes time to work out all of the bugs in the system, and it still may not do what it needs to do, but you have a bumper!

With the increase of multiple systems also comes an increased risk to you for errors. In a multiple system application, an order that is placed in the EMR system for a blood transfusion has to "cross over" to the Lab's system. When this does not occur, the patient does not receive the treatment in a timely fashion or maybe not at all. The problem is often discovered when the physician finds the hemoglobin level still low the next day and questions the nurse about the transfusion order. Safety measures are usually in place to insure that the orders are carried out, but they do occur. Ask if the hospital uses individual computer programs in their ancillary departments and how long they have been integrated. It is possible that the hospital systems have not been integrated, which also causes more confusion and may require practitioners to document in more than one systems. Orders can get "lost" or may not cross over with efficient integrations, so ask what system applications are used in the various areas of the hospital, and if they are integrated.

EMR and the Nurse

There are many things that the nurse does for the patient and with the EMR and the nurse is expected to utilize the computer more now than ever before. The buzz words for nurses across this country are "relationship based care". Sounds like a really good concept, but the bottom line is that we are continuing to ask more and more of nurses with an already over worked and under staffed workforce.

A friend told me the other day she had got a call at 5:00 AM from her hospital to see if she could come into work for the day. She told them that she had a class from 8:00-10:00 AM at the hospital, but that she could work after that. She went directly to the floor after the class and was suppose to work until 4:00 PM, but ending up staying until 8:00 PM because of staffing needs, then was asked if she could stay until 11:00 PM. Short handed + over worked staff = errors. Every year there are at least 1.5 million patients that are harmed due to errors, and there are many more that go unreported. The EMR can be both an answer to this problem, and also a causation of medical errors. Studies have shown that computerized charting on the EMR can require more time that could have been spent with patients. Working with computers in a clinical setting can take more time if done properly and there are only so many hours in a day. Nurses are often faced with the difficult task of taking care of the patients or having great looking documentation.

The nurse to patient ratios have not changed, and may have even gone up at some facilities, as we also ask the nurse to spend more time documenting in the computer. Some hospitals that have placed a high priority on patient safety have implemented as low as 4:1 patient to nurse ratios on their regular medical units. If you are a patient, ask your nurse how many patients she has that day, as first hand experience is more relevant than you asking the hospital. No hospital wants to tell you that their night shift nurse had 10 patients last night because they did not have enough nurses scheduled. Many nurses struggle with providing the patient with adequate care while meeting the hospital requirements for documentation, but the hospitals that find this balance are the ones with happy nurses and grateful patients. I had a manager tell me that nurses should not discuss the number of patients they are responsible for with the patients, but patients know if the nurse has quality time to spend with them, without the nurse ever uttering a word.

You also need to ask your family and friends that have been to your local hospital if the nursing staff spent adequate time with them, or if they were just a number on her list. Nurses are point of care providers, as they are often the first to greet the patient when they arrive to the unit and the last one to provide the discharge instructions. Nurses are the last to review the medications before administration and are often the first to see the labs. We just need to make sure that the expectation of the EMR coupled with the number of patients does not put the patient at risk.

Allergic Reactions

Most computerized systems offer electronic monitoring of allergies. If a medication is ordered that the patient is allergic to, an alert should be generated. These alerts are great, but when it occurs, someone is still required to make a decision. Should it be "ordered anyway" or should the physician change the order. If the pharmacist gets the alert, they are subject to becoming alert fatigue as they could see hundreds of these alerts every day, and could bypass something that should not have been allowed for the patient.

I see some nurses relying on the computer to a point where they do not look at the medications in the same manner as they did when it was on paper. Because the computer has this medication listed for the patient, it must be safe to administer, right? We have taken away some of the critical thinking and replaced it with trust in a computerized system that is unable to think critically.

As a patient, it is important for you to know the medications that are being administered, even if you must write them down along with the times for administration. Ask the nurse what medication she is giving you and the dosages. You just need to be proactive in your treatment plan, which includes being informed, and holding the clinicians accountable. Ask your nurse if your allergies are listed in the computer as this is your first line of defense. Also, make sure they know what happened when you reacted to the medication and have it recorded in the computer for easy access.

We had notified Senior Citizens from our local community that we would enter their allergies and medications into our computer system if they would provide us with the information. This is great information to have in the computer when an emergency occurs. Even though medications can change, it is a quick reference, and can be verified in a shorter amount of time.

One patient sent in three whole pages of "allergies" to medications, at least by her standards. The patient listed such things as Morphine makes her weak in the knees, or Benadryl makes her sleepy. You need to understand that these are simply side effects of the drug and are not truly classified as allergies. Although allergic reactions can vary from minor annoying symptoms, they can also cause life-threatening situations. If you are unsure if you have an allergy or side effect to a medication, ask your nurse or physician for assistance. Allergies, along with the type of reaction, should be listed and easily assessable in every electronic medical record.

Phone Orders

Hospitals across the nation are also faced with the increased number of "phone orders" to the nurse since they have implemented the EMR. This requires time and action on the nurse's part, since the physician did not do their part. Some physicians admit that they go see their patients, then call the floor on their way to the office and give verbal orders to the nurse.

So here may be your scenario: Your physician just visited 10 patients at the hospital, all with different conditions, on different units and nurses. He did not put any orders in the computer, but has to call each nurse and give a "verbal order" for each patient. Sound a little scary? It should, as verbal orders can also increase your risk for medical errors. If your physician is entering your orders there can be great advantages and a safety element as well.

One great advantage of the EMR is the ability to read the orders. I have gathered around a chart with several other nurses trying to "read" what the doctor has written for an order. We would all chime in with our "interpretation", and if consensus could not be reached, the doctor would be called. Gone are the days of unintelligible writing with the implementation of the EMR order entry. There are some EMR systems that utilize voice activated technology with relatively high accuracy, but can be a big luxury that many hospitals have not purchased. The biggest downfall for voice activated systems is the language barrier, but that has been a minuet problem for most systems.

Phone orders are sometimes necessary as the physicians do not have access to a computer, but you need to know if your physicians place their own orders. Direct order placement reduces your risk for error, so let your physician know that this is important to you.

Privacy Anyone?

With the integration of the EMR also comes a privacy issue. Do you know who has access to your medical records? You might say it is only your nurse and your physician, but the circle is much bigger, and the regulation of this information is not always a high priority. Remember, for many hospitals, this is a new road that they are building from the ground up and most of their focus is on just keeping the programs running.

I compare it to building a road without a great foundation if they do not have security measures in mind. For those of us that live in the northern states, we know all too well that "potholes" occur when we do not have an adequate foundation. All of the care-providers at the hospital, the unit clerks, medical records, finance, the lab departments, the physician and most of the staff in their office have access to your medical information. The hospital gives the "speech" for confidentially, but what are they actually doing to monitor it? Personal information should be just that; personal. Criminals are always looking for new ways to collect information that could be used in a malicious manner, and many EMR's contain that type of information. Recently a hospital in Indiana had good intentions for protecting the patient information, but when they started providing the patient with an online bill paying service, they left the system unprotected from hackers. They could not tell the hospital patrons if anyone stole their information, they could only say that someone might have taken it. The hospital will provide free credit checks for a year, but security measures need to be in place to prevent it from occurring to begin with. The government wants this electronic record, but there also needs to be regulations that protect the patient. Some hospitals do a better job of protecting your information than others, but you still have a right to know who has been given access to your records.

Patient Safety

The EMR is more than just your average computer program, there are patient's lives at risk. This is not one area you want someone "practicing", as it could be a life or death situation. For your safety, the hospital needs to have "key" people, with hospital experience, in leadership roles. When you have someone that understands medical terminology, treatments and process in this key role, the hospital can have a wonderful system. It is ok to ask about the IT department and the credentials for the top executives in that area as well. The risks associated with patient care are much greater in a hospital setting, so the hospital should be placing a high priority on finding employees with both clinical and computer experience. You might also want to know how long they have been with the hospital, or if they are a contracted service. Just because you can ride a bike, does not mean you can drive a car, so make a thorough investigation.

Ask what computerized system they are using and what safety measures are in place to protect the patient from errors. Inquire about the type of training the clinicians and ancillary staff received in preparation of the computerized system, and what programs the hospital has in place to keep the staff up to date on system changes and upgrades.

For those facilities that just "pull the paper", I suggest that you think back to what it was like the first time you drove a car. As with anything new, there is a time of adjustment, no, I should say a BIG time of adjustment. You not only have the new orders being put into the computer (which is new to the clinical staff), but then all of the orders need to go to the right place, at the right time, and say the right thing. The physicians, pharmacy, laboratory, respiratory therapist, blood bank, physical therapy, dietary, admitting, and nursing (just to name a few) all need to receive the orders in the proper manner at the correct time.

In nursing we have the 5 rights…Right medication, right dose, right patient, right time and right route. The EMR also has to function properly and it is the responsibility of the hospital to make sure it is right from the start. Unless you signed up to be a "guinea pig" when you arrived at the hospital, ask questions about the electronic record and how it pertains to your care.

Considerations for the EMR:
1. Find out if your hospital has an EMR that is currently being utilized.
2. If they do have an EMR, how long has computerized order entry been in use?
3. Do they plan any system upgrades or improvements?
4. On what date will the system be upgraded?
5. How many different computerized systems does the hospital have and are they integrated with each other?
6. How much training did the clinicians have for the EMR?
7. Make sure your allergies are documented in the computer system along with the reaction.
8. Find out who enters the orders into the computer.
9. If the physicians are required to do this, find out how computer savvy your doctor is.
10. Ask your physician how he utilizes phone orders.
11. Ask your nurse what the medication is and the dose prior to administration, every time.
12. Find out what the nurse to patient ratio is for all units. Intensive care units have different ratios than the regular medical units. There may also be a different ratio for the day shift verses the night shift.
13. Ask how your confidential information is handled and who has access to it.
14. If internet access is given to your medical record, you need to know what safety measures are in place to protect it.
15. Ask how long the executive level employees that are managing the EMR have been in a clinical setting.

Hospital Evaluation Chart

Questions for hospital evaluation	Hospital
How many beds does the hospital have?	
Is the hospital a teaching facility?	
If it is a teaching hospital, what schools do they partner with?	
How many residents do they have at the hospital?	
How many medical students and interns do they have?	
What specialties (Surgery, OB/GYN, etc) have residents?	
What diagnostic equipment do they have on site?	
What types of Specialist are on staff 24/7?	
Are the ancillary depts. (like Endo and MRI) staffed 24/7?	
What is the hospital's infection rate?	
Does the hospital see enough patients to report for the CMS information?	
What areas does the hospital not meet the required reporting for the CMS?	
Are the results of the CMS and JCAHO reports positive?	
Did surgical patients receive antibiotics within 1 hour of their surgical incision?	

SURVIVING YOUR MEDICAL CRISIS

Did heart attack patients receive necessary treatments?	
Has there been any sentinel events at this hospital?	
Are they JCACHO or AOA approved?	
What is the hospital's mortality rate on the CMS reports?	
What is the rating given to physicians and nurses from the patients?	
Do the patients find the rooms clean?	
Was the patient's pain controlled?	
Is the hospital a Center of Excellence?	
What specialties have been recognized as a Center of Excellence?	
Are the rooms private or semi-private?	
Your thoughts after personally visiting the hospital?	
How many miles is this hospital from your home?	
Does your physician have privileges to practice at this hospital?	
Is the hospital participating in clinical studies?	
What physicians are participating in research at this time?	
Check the financial status of the hospital.	

Does the hospital accept your insurance?	
Does the hospital treat patients that do not have insurance?	

CHAPTER 2

How to Find the Best Physicians for Your Care

Finding the right physician could be as difficult as finding the right mate. You need someone that is not only compatible with you, but someone that wants a relationship for a long time. This chapter covers some basic information for those that would like to locate a physician on their own, but if you would like to have someone else do the research for you, go to www.MyMedicalAdvisor.net. This site provides you with physicians and hospitals that match your preferences for quality of care. There is a fee associated with this service, but it is well worth it if you do not have the time for your own research.

If you have ever moved to a new city, or had a baby, you may have had the experience of trying to find a new doctor. If you are like most people, you have asked your neighbors or coworkers who they have for a physician. Some insurance plans may even dictate who you can see, or you just picked a name out of the phone book. There are certain criteria that my physicians have to meet, but your standards may be different from mine. No matter what method you use for finding the "perfect physician", you need to understand a little bit about their different medical degrees and specialties.

A Medical Doctor (MD) and a Doctor of Osteopathic Medicine (DO) have very similar training. Both types of doctors have gone through a 4 year undergraduate degree program, taken the MCAT, and completed a 3-7 year residency program. They take different licensing exams, but must pass the exam in order to practice medicine, according to state licensing boards. M.D.'s and D.O.'s treat the same kinds of patients and use the same tools and treatment methods. The main difference is the D.O.'s have received training to perform osteopathic manipulations on the patients. They tend to focus on the "whole person" and preventative care. This is not to say that your M.D. does not focus on the whole person, it just means that the D.O. has additional training in this area.

D.O.'s tend to practice primarily in family practice, pediatrics or internal medicine, but can be found in all specialties. There are not as many Osteopathic Medical schools in the U.S., so we tend to see more M.D.'s in the clinical setting, but most hospitals grant privileges to both types of doctors. No matter what degree the physicians have after their name, they have different functioning methods for their individual practices.

A few months after I moved to Michigan, I found out that I was pregnant. Finding a physician was a little tricky as I really did not want to make any "grand" announcements until I saw the physician, so my inquiry needed to be conducted in a discreet manner. I was fortunate that my sister-in-law worked for a physician's group, so her first question was, did I want a physician in an individual or group practice. This is one of the first things you must decide, as both single practices and multi-physician practices have benefits. The bottom line is, if you select a group, you need to feel comfortable with everyone in the practice. You may never have to see one of the other physicians, but there is that chance. Doctors work long hours and also need time off. Those practicing in a multi-physician setting often can provide the best care when they are covering for another physician as they have access to office records, and direct contact if necessary with your primary physician, even though they may not be on-call.

Even if you select an individual practice, they will still have someone cover for them when they are gone. I had selected an individual for my OB/GYN and three days before I gave birth, I had to see another physician at the hospital because my physician was on vacation. So make sure to ask you physician who will take care of you when they are not available, and try to meet that physician as well.

Physician Specialties

Physicians can specialize in various areas of medicine. With this type of insurance plan, the physician receives a specific amount of money for your care, which could discourage the primary care physician from referring you to a specialist. Some insurance plans pay the physician a specific amount of money for your care, which could discourage the primary care physician to refer you to a specialist. If he refers you to a specialist, he does not get paid like he would if he was the one treating you.

With physicians specializing in all different areas of medicine, it is possible that you could have several on your healthcare team at one time. The key component with numerous physicians treating your condition is communication, as they all need to be on the same page. If your specialist recommends treatment for your condition, without knowing what medications the other physician has prescribed, you could be putting your health at risk. They need to communicate with each other, and you need to inform them of all treatments being administered.

In the clinical setting you can often find physicians recommending other physicians that they "like". It reminds me of children playing in the sand box. You are "allowed" in the sandbox if the leader of the gang likes you, or if you know the right people. The "you scratch my back and I'll scratch yours", scenario can also come into play in the clinical setting. You need to be aware that this goes on, and make sure that the physicians that are being recommended to you are qualified, and meet or exceed your standards of care.

Just because a specialist is recommended to you by another physician, does not mean that you are not allowed to request someone else. Remember you are part of the decision making team, and hopefully you have your "list" of preferred doctors already developed, before you need them. I have had many patients tell me

SURVIVING YOUR MEDICAL CRISIS

that they are unhappy with a physician, and there is absolutely no reason for you not to be pleased with the care you are receiving. If there is just a personality conflict, you need to weigh that issue against the physician's experience, and skills. A woman came to me when my husband had a brain tumor and she expressed a conflict that she had with our Neurosurgeon. When I probed a little deeper, it was just a personality conflict between the two. At that point, we had not had any problems with the surgeon, and his qualifications were impeccable.

We decided that it didn't matter much to us if the physician was "warm and fuzzy" if he did not know how to remove my husband's brain tumor. A nice bedside manor is always a plus, but they better know what they are doing first and foremost. Some of the websites listed later in this chapter allows you to compare specialist in your area, as well as the number of years they have been practicing, but gather your list for future availability.

Specialist	Physician's Name
General Surgeon	
Pulmonologist (Respiratory)	
Neurologist (Nerves/Brain issues)	
Orthopedic (Bones)	
Cardiologist (Heart-Circulatory)	
Hematologist/Oncologist (Blood-Cancer)	
Nephrologists/Urologist (Kidney)	
Pediatrics (Children/Babies)	

Your primary care physician should be able to make recommendations for specialized physicians, but this is only your starting point. Do your research of the websites, and talk to your family and friends, and then draw your conclusions. If you have this list when you are faced with an emergency, you come prepared and this can give you peace of mind about your care providers.

Health Insurance

Your insurance may determine who you can see and when, but you need to take an active part in finding out what physicians are available to you. Most insurance companies offer a listing of physicians that participate with their insurance plan, but I would never let that be my only determining factor for seeing a certain physician. Just because they participate does not mean that they are a "good" physician. Sometimes it just comes down to the fact that they are not "right" for you. I have had patients tell me that they want a physician that "speaks English". I am not saying this in any prejudice manner, but if you cannot understand your physician, no matter what language you speak, your risk for errors goes up.

Communication is an important element for any relationship, but is essential in a patient-doctor relationship. My best recommendation would be to first ask family, friends and coworkers who they would refer you to. It would be even better if you can ask those that work with the physicians for a referral. The healthcare providers work with the physicians daily and know how they treat their patients. This personal evaluation is always beneficial when seeking a new physician.

I used to joke with my husband and say "that doctor is on the do not let him touch me list". There is some validity to this, and as clinicians, we have an understanding of what needs to be done for certain conditions or diseases. We see what tests the physicians order, treatment plans, and then we see the results. We recognize those physicians that have a record for impeccable care, because they stand out. If your insurance dictates who you can see, you might not have these reputable physicians accessible to you, or it might cost you more if they provide your care.

One surgeon comes to mind when I think about impeccable care, which also set the standard for everyone else taking care of her patients. The nurses all knew what her expectations were, and if the patient was not treated to her standards of care, you heard about it! She wanted the best for her patients and she insisted that all the healthcare providers were on the "same team".

Physicians are human, and believe it or not, they make mistakes too, but the nurses know the good ones. I also like the recommendations of physicians that I trust. When I needed a new OB/GYN after mine retired, I asked a physician friend who he sends his wife to. I later found out that this same OB/GYN physician my friend had recommended was also the doctor that a lot of nurses have as their physician.

When you gain the respect of those that you work with, it says a lot about your capabilities and bedside manner. When you work with physicians all the time, you get to see first hand their successes, along with their failures. You understand how they feel about their patients, and those on the medical team. Physicians are also known by the fruits of their labor, but those that work by their side, often know them the best.

Proactive Healthcare

Most people wait until they are faced with a difficult situation before they meet a specialist. Just like any good parent would want to know about the 18 year old boy that is taking their 16 year old daughter out on a date, you need to find out about the physician that is making decisions about your life. It is ok to ask how many cases like yours they have taken care of or how many surgeries they have performed. You should also ask what their infection rate is and how many years they have been practicing. Ask if they are open to alternative treatments and how they think they could help your condition.

You can gather a wealth of information when you ask these questions. Not only will you get the answers, but you can also see how the physician reacts to the questions, and his bedside manner. In essence, you are "hiring" a new physician, and every good employer has questions for the prospective employee, so go prepared. If the physician does not like being questioned, that also sends loud messages. Sometimes it is good to also look at websites and listen to what other patients have had to say.

HealthGrades website and the "Five-Star Doctors"

University students have become very "wise" students if they have utilized the websites that "rate the professor". They can find out all kinds of information, and generally it is pretty accurate. Healthcare is starting to follow suit, as consumers become more conscious about their healthcare. Your online research should consist of several different sites, and new ones are popping up every day. The CMS information can be found on the website: (http://www.hospitalcompare.hhs.gov

No physician is perfect, but they should be striving for that and it should show in the reported information. The CMS site is free and provides excellent information about the physician, but www.healthgrades.com also provides information about the hospital and your local physicians. There are also other websites available that allow you to write comments or provide feedback about your physician's care. The combination of the sites can give you a pretty good picture of your local hospitals and physicians. Information on sites that collect patient's feedback should not be the sole basis for your decision when finding a doctor, but it should have an impact on your decision making process. The downside to some of the websites is the lack of information for some physicians, but for those that are on the list, they generally reflect accurate information for the physicians.

Before I knew about the online ratings, we saw a physician for my husband's hip. We had been told years ago that he would need a hip replacement, and he had been experiencing a lot of pain, so we decided to go see someone new. Since the physician that had originally made the diagnosis had retired, we checked around, and went off a recommendation of a friend who is a nurse. After our initial visit, we were not impressed with the physician. His ability or lack there of, to answer our questions was not up to par with our standards, and later when I was writing this book I read several reviews for this orthopedic specialist that all concurred! We did not pursue any replacement with that physician but after reading the comments on the rating site, we just knew we had made the right decision. The hospital that this surgeon practiced at, had a very low infection rate, but the physician did not meet our standards. When it comes to your care, you want to have the best of both worlds if possible.

You must remember the old adage that when someone is not happy with their treatment, they tell 10 others, but if they ARE happy with the treatment they only tell one to two other individuals. You need to consider what the website says, but that is only one factor in the equation.

It is nice to have all of this information in one place, but can be a little overwhelming for those that are not computer literate, so let's start by doing a search for a physician.

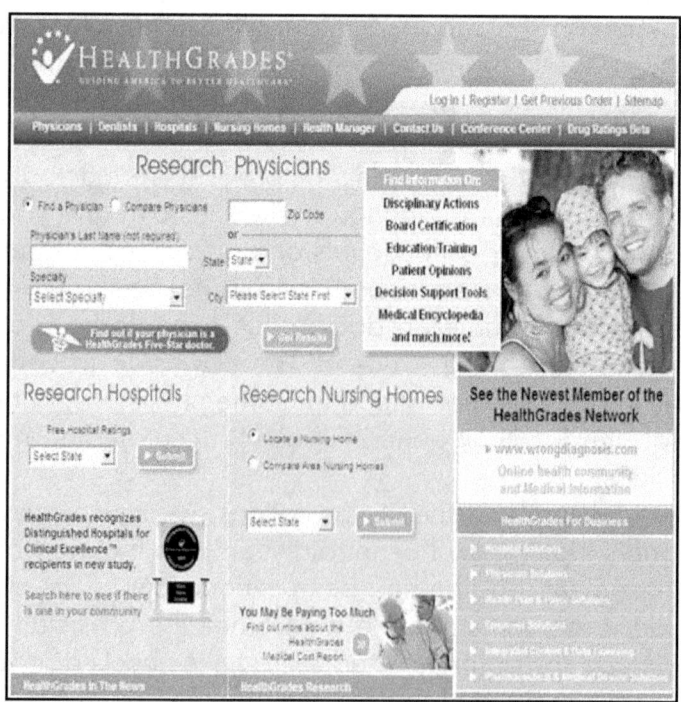

(Illustration 6) Used by permission of Healthgrades.com

HOW TO FIND THE BEST PHYSICIANS FOR YOUR CARE

In *illustration 6* you will see that the button in the upper left hand corner is preselected to "Find a Physician". You can further your search by selecting a specialty along with a City and State, or a Zip Code. If you know the physician's name, you can narrow your search even further. If you conducted a general search, a list of all the area physicians in that City and Specialty you selected will be displayed.

Illustration 7 shows the results from a general search for a Cardiologist in Mt. Vernon, Ohio.

Physician Results

For each physician listed below, the first report is only $12.95 and $9.95 for each additional Physician Quality Report on this order only.*

Name	Location	Specialty	Gender
Debbra L Debaets, MD	Mount Vernon, OH	Cardiology	Female
Barry S George, MD	Mount Vernon, OH	Cardiology	Male
Arsad Karcic, MD	Mount Vernon, OH	Cardiology	Male
Timothy P Obarski, DO	Mount Vernon, OH	Cardiology	Male
Jawahar Palaniappan, MD	Mount Vernon, OH	Cardiology	Male
Joseph R Poole Jr, MD	Mount Vernon, OH	Cardiology	Male
Gangaram Rasa, MD	Mount Vernon, OH	Cardiology	Male
Tribeni N Srivastava, MD	Mount Vernon, OH	Cardiology	Male
Ruben Trono, MD	Mount Vernon, OH	Cardiology	Male

(Illustration 7) Used by permission of Healthgrades.com

If you are just looking to find who the cardiologists are around you, this part is free. By just clicking on the name of the physician, you can see general information listed on each of the tabs; including a Physician Profile, Patient Ratings and if they are in a group practice.

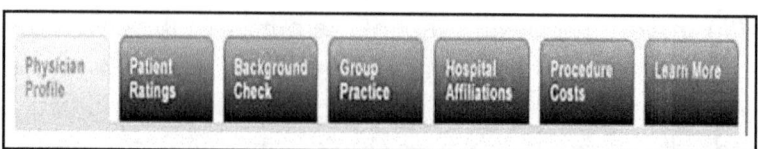

Used by permission of Healthgrades.com

This also can let you know what hospitals the physician is affiliated with and the individual hospital ratings. If you would like more detailed information such as a background check, board certifications, Five-Star Recognition and much more, it will cost you $12.95 for the first physician and $9.95 for any additional doctor.

HealthGrades states on their website that their "5 Star Doctors are affiliated with a hospital that is highly rated by HealthGrades; are board certified in the specialty they practice; have never had their license restricted or revoked; are free of state or federal disciplinary actions; and are free of any malpractice claims. Receiving quality healthcare can help you effectively manage your condition and recover more quickly when you are ill. By pairing a high quality hospital with a highly skilled physician, your chances of quality care should also be higher.

HealthGrades will provide you with the physician's: location, map to office, specialty, medical school, residency location, gender and years since graduation. Where the physician had their training does matter, as medical schools are very selective about whom they accept, and those with the best reputations are not going to take just anyone. It does not mean that they are guaranteed to have more educational experiences to various diseases and conditions at reputable institutions, but the chances are greater at the larger hospitals as they will have a larger patient population.

Bedside manner is also rated on the website and can be very influential when selecting a physician, so you want to know what others have to say. HealthGrades.com and ratemydoctor.com show what previous patients have said, and provides national average comparisons. The doctor's punctuality, how soon could you make an appointment, friendliness of the staff, etc., are all things provided on these sites. If you are not a person that likes to "wait" for an hour before you see the doctor, and the ratings say it was just that, you might need to consider if this physician is a good fit for you. The positive ratings need to be weighed against the negatives and see where the physician comes out.

Disciplinary Actions

In the detailed report, HealthGrades also tells you if the physician has had any disciplinary actions taken against him. Most medical boards do not take this action lightly. Disciplinary action usually results if the physician has been formally charged with doing something wrong, including any felony charges that may not even be related to his medical practice. Information is usually turned over to the board if a hospital has taken disciplinary actions that have resulted in the physician's termination, or hospital privileges being revoked, as disciplinary measures. Most malpractice judgments will also be reported to the licensing board. The downside to some of the websites is that the reporting is only for the last 5 years. This may be extended as the years go by since the reporting is so new on the websites. Disciplinary information is available through each state, but it can be very cumbersome to locate. HealthGrades makes this information easy to find. Another site that provides this information is http://www.choicetrust.com. At HealthPulse (choicetrust.com) you will be able to buy a day pass for $11.95 or a single report for $7.95. This is very reasonable as you can search all day for one low price. It will provide some of the same information most other sites will provide including if there has been any disciplinary actions taken against this physician.

Proactive Healthcare

Doing your research a head of time can prevent headaches later, but what you can do if you are in the hospital, and do not want the physician you have? This can be a little tricky, depending on the situation. I had a family member come to my office one day in tears and wanted to know if I could help her get her mother out of the hospital. Her mother had come to that hospital because "Dr.

Joe" worked there and he had come so highly recommended by her friends. The patient's condition had not improved since her surgery, and had actually taken a turn for the worse. The difficult equation to figure out in this type of situation is if the problem is "Dr Joe's" fault, or is it the patient's response to the treatment.

Just because things are not going "right" does not mean that the physician has done something wrong. The patient and her daughter felt that they were not getting the answers that they needed and that things just kept "going wrong". I was able to contact "Dr. Joe" for the patient and explain the situation. With this small intervention, the daughter was already starting to feel better. The physician had no idea that the patient felt that way, so he came immediately to answer their questions, and discuss the disease process more in depth. This did not instantly "heal" the patient, but it did take away some of the resentment that had developed due to the patient's poor recovery. When you think your condition is someone else's fault, it creates bitterness and interferes with your mental wellbeing. You need to have all of the facts about your condition before you pass judgment on your physician, but this might require you taking an active role in your treatment.

Our bodies are very complex and things do not always go as planned. There are many physicians that loose sleep over their patient's condition, so make sure you communicate effective with your physician about your thoughts, feelings and expectations. Remember that they are not mind readers, but no matter how many years of education or training they might have, they still are working for you.

Transfer to another hospital

Transfer to another facility can be a process that can take time. First you must find a physician at another hospital that will accept your case. This would be a little like the "new" physician (at the other hospital) buying a car from the local transmission shop with a blown transmission for the third time. If you are hospitalized, there are obvious risks associated with your case, not only for the "new" physician, but also for you.

If you are transferring because you do not like the care you have received, the "new" physician may also be a little concerned that you may not be "happy" with him either. Once a physician has been located, you must now wait for a bed at the other hospital. Depending on your condition and bed availability, I have seen this take several days, even for critical patients. Many hospitals these days run near capacity and they must also account for the people they have in their emergency rooms as well. If you are being transferred just because you need a different level of care than what your current hospital can offer, physicians are more eager to accept your case.

You will usually have an ambulance or helicopter for the transfer, depending on where you are going, and you should check with your insurance to see if this will be covered, or you might be surprised later when the bill arrives.

If you have issues with the staff or nurses at the hospital, you need to ask for the unit manager. They should be able to resolve any issues, but you can also ask for the risk manager or patient advocate at the hospital, for those unresolved issues. Their job is to act as a mediator for you or your loved one.

Many issues can be prevented by just doing your "homework" and knowing in advance, what doctors and hospitals meet your standards of care. Most patients end up at a hospital near their home, but if you are out of town, you may not have a lot of choices. You might end of getting whoever is "on call" for that day, so just remember that you are not forced to have this doctor if there is a problem.

Hospital Affiliations

Even though you are selecting the physician, you also need to consider where they work. I spoke earlier about the CMS reports, but you can see how they compare to local and national hospitals on the HealthGrades website as well. Being able to see the hospital's area of expertise may direct your selection for a physician. You stand

◄ SURVIVING YOUR MEDICAL CRISIS

the best chance of getting the care you need if you go to the hospital that specializes in that area.

Search the reports and know the specialties that each hospital ranks highly in. Some hospital ratings show that the hospital does not "rank" for a particular clinical area of service. This may be cause for alarm, as the hospital may not be treating enough patients in this area for reporting measures.

In *graph 8* you can see that Hospital #1 has mostly "5 Star ratings" which are above average for the specific clinical service area. The "3 star ratings" indicate that the hospital is performing as expected, and the dot indicates that information is not reported. The hospitals receive the ratings because of the services they are providing. No hospital is perfect, but "5 Stars" looks like they are working really hard at achieving that perfection.

Clinical Service Area	Hospital # 1	Hospital # 2	Hospital # 3
	►Full Report	►Full Report	►Full Report
Cardiac	★★★★★	●	★★★
Critical Care	★★★	●	★★★
Gastrointestinal	★★★★★	●	★★★
General Surgery	●	●	●
Orthopedic	★★★	●	★★★
Pulmonary	★★★★★	★★★★★	★★★★★
Stroke	★★★★★	★★★	★★★
Vascular	★★★★★	●	★★★

Illustration 9 *(Used by permission of Healthgrades.com)*

There are other websites that provide information about doctors and some are even free. Here are a few to look over:

http://www.MyMedicalAdvisor.Net
http://www.ratemds.com/social/
http://www.drscore.com/about/faqs.cfm
http://www.vimo.com/doctor/doctorreviewsall.php

http://www.physicianreports.com
http://www.vitals.com

How to find the right Physician

Here are some general questions that you need answered in order to find the physician that is right for you:

1. Is the physician a Medical Doctor (MD) or a Doctor of Osteopathy (DO)?
2. Are they in a group or individual practice?
3. Who covers for them when they are gone?
4. What types of insurance do they accept?
5. How long have they been practicing?
6. What is their area of specialty?
7. Where did they go to medical school and perform their residency?
8. What are their office hours?
9. Where are they located?
10. What hospitals do they have privileges at?
11. If you wanted an appointment, how soon would you be able to see them?
12. Is it a male or female?
13. What types of services do they offer in their office (x-ray, lab, etc)?
14. What awards or recognitions have they received?
15. What languages does the physician speak, and what is their primary language?
16. What ratings does the physician receive on HealthGrades or other websites?
17. How many patients do they see each day in their office?
18. What do other patients have to say about the physician?
19. Does the physician practice at a hospital that meets your standards of care?
20. Has the physician ever had any disciplinary actions taken against them?
21. Who recommends this physician?

CHAPTER 3

Understanding Your Disease Could Save Your Life

Disease can be defined as a disorder or an ineffectively functioning of a body system, organ, part or structure. Though your condition could be a result of various causative agents, the bottom line is, something is wrong with you. Unless you spend a lot of time at the hospital or have relatives with chronic diseases, certain medical conditions may be unfamiliar to you. It is important for you be your own best advocate, by taking the initiative in your health promotion, as well as the treatment process.

When my sister was diagnosed with cancer, she wanted to know about the disease and how it should be diagnosed, as well as the treatment options. Patients often lack the knowledge of what diagnostic tests should be done for their condition; let alone what the results should be. Prevention of disease or knowing when to see a doctor can play a key role in you recovery process.

As an important part of your healthcare team, you need to be informed, and the best way to accomplish that task is by researching the disease or condition. There have been entire books written about

◄ SURVIVING YOUR MEDICAL CRISIS

just one of the disease listed in this book, so this information is meant to be a stepping stone, which provides basic concepts about diseases you could experience.

Over the next few pages, a brief description of the most common conditions that bring patients into the hospital will be covered. Once you have a diagnosis, you need to understand what the disease is, what caused it, and then what to expect for treatment. Medical conditions can be very complex, as our bodies are so unique, but some standards can apply. The basic treatments will also be covered to provide a general consideration for what to expect while at the hospital. A clear understanding of the disease can assist in your decision making process as you will be an informed part of the medical team.

Acute Myocardial Infarction (AMI)

This is a long way of saying that you have had what is more commonly known as a heart attack. There are many blood vessels in your heart and one or more of them has been blocked which prevented the necessary blood to flow to that area. Most AMIs are caused by a plaque buildup in your arteries, which can aid in a clot formation, which can result in the artery being closed off. Without this blood supply to the heart, the tissue can die, leading to heart damage or even death. Conditions that can put you at higher risk for a heart attack include high blood pressure and high cholesterol. If you get regular health screenings, these conditions can be discovered early, but for those that do not even know that they have these risk factors, they may have a time bomb waiting to go off.

Symptoms

Signs and Symptoms of an AMI usually start out slow with mild discomfort or pain in the chest. Patients can experience pain that radiates in one or both arms, in the neck, jaw or back. Women often present with atypical symptoms so they are more at risk of being misdiagnosed. Woman may be more likely to report shortness of breath, back or jaw pain, nausea and vomiting. If the chest pain is mistaken for heartburn, the patient will often dismiss the symptoms, which delays treatment. If you feel like you have an elephant sitting on your chest, or any other of the symptoms listed, you need to be seen by a healthcare professional immediately.

Chest pain warrants a call to 911 emergency services as you want to be the #1 priority when you come through those hospital doors, and you also want to be in the hands of people that are trained to treat this condition on the way to the hospital.

Upon arrival to the hospital, you should receive immediate attention where an assessment and treatment should be initiated. Blood work should show an elevated troponin level if you really are having a heart attack. In *Graph 5* you will be able to see the normal lab tests that are done when a heart attack is suspected, along with the normal range for each test.

Expect to have a specialized physician in cardiac issues, called a Cardiologist, who will evaluate your condition. If you know of a doctor you would like to see, this is the time to make that request. If you do not know any doctors, you should see the section of this book on physicians. If the diagnosis is confirmed, you are usually admitted to a coronary care unit for at least the first 36 hours to allow those that specialize in cardiac issues to monitor your condition.

Treatment Plan

Some or all of the following diagnostic tests and treatments could be initiated when the physician suspects a diagnosis of an AMI:

> Blood Tests: CBC, Chem 12, Troponin, D-Dimer
> Coronary Angiogram
> High resolution chest CT scan
> ECG (Electrocardiography)
> Antiplatelet Agents (Plavix)
> Supplemental Oxygen
> Nitrates
> Beta-Blockers (Tenormin, Toprol, Lopressor, etc)

Blood thinners
Fibrinolytics
Surgical Bypass
Angiotensin Converting Enzyme Inhibitors
(ACE Inhibitors)
Cardiac Stress Test
Implantable Cardiac Defibrillators
Cardiac Rehabilitation
t-PA
Balloon Angioplasty
Stent placement

One cardiologist gave me the acronym of "MONA" to treat someone with a heart attack. It stands for:

M- Morphine which helps with the pain and also the heart function.
O- Oxygen to increase the levels in the blood.
N- Nitroglycerine dilates the blood vessels to improve blood flow.
A- Aspirin reduces the inflammation and clotting activity.

There are other treatments that can be provided, but these are the basics. You should also be given a beta-blocker and possibly a drug like t-PA that will be administered to help dissolve the clot. Emergency angioplasty or surgery may also be required to remove the clot. There are treatments that can be performed that can save your life, so it is important that you do not over-look the symptoms of a heart attack, and seek immediate attention. Your heart should be constantly monitored with an electrocardiogram machine which can show any new abnormalities. Depending on your condition you could be out of the hospital in just a few days. Life style modification such as diet and exercise should be discussed with your physician. Cardiac rehab may be necessary to regain your strength and endurance after experiencing a heart attack, but should be tailored to your physical condition.

Cardio Pulmonary Resuscitation (CPR)

One more important topic we must cover is Cardiopulmonary

Resuscitation (CPR). When a heart attack occurs, the blood stops pumping through the heart, and if you know CPR, you can buy precious time that could save someone's life.

When I was 12 years old, we received a call from my Uncle Bill who had been working with my Grandfather that day on the farm. He said that my Grandfather had collapsed, and the only thing he knew to do was call 911 for an ambulance, which was about 15-20 minutes away. My Mother and I got in the car immediately and actually arrived at the farm before the emergency squad, but it was too late. My Grandfather was gone. Had Uncle Bill known CPR, Grandpa might still be alive today. Your local fire station, hospital or community center should be able to tell you where you can take a CPR class. You never know when something like this will happen, or whose life you could save, so take a class.

A few websites to research heart attacks are:

http://www.clevelandclinicmeded.com/medicalpubs/diseasemanagement/cardiology/acutemi/acutemi.htm
http://www.americanheart.org
http://www.webmd.com

Bone Fractures

A fracture occurs when there is a break in any bone in your body. Most patients seen in the hospital with a fracture either come from auto accidents, or a fall, but they can be caused from other conditions such as cancer or osteoporosis. There are many types of fractures, ranging from a hairline fracture that can be hard to see even on an X-ray, to a compound fracture where the bone has come through the skin.

Signs and Symptoms

Fractures hurt because the nerves surrounding the broken bone become irritated. Fractures often experience bleeding and swelling which also can result in pain. In some cases the muscles surrounding the broken bone can spasm, resulting in extreme pain. Most fractures are easy to detect because you can see the obvious deformity of the affected body part. When our daughter had a broken nose after taking an elbow during a basketball game, there was no question if it was broke. The bridge of her nose did not form a straight line. In some cases, the signs and symptoms can give a good indication of the condition.

Location of the fracture can determine the signs and symptoms you will experience. You may experience loss of movement, pain, swelling and bruising. If the fracture is a compound fracture, it is very evident, since the bone is through the skin. There can be some visual deformity, with one leg being shorter or it may just look "out of place". An X-ray will usually provide the confirmed diagnosis and will show the exact location and type of fracture.

Treatment

If you think a fracture has occurred, try to immobilize it until help arrives. Try not to use the affected area as it can cause further aggravation or damage. Ice packs can reduce the swelling often associated with a fracture.

The physician may be able to put the bone back into proper alignment and hold it into place with a cast in an office setting. Most complex fractures require surgery to put the bones back into proper alignment, and may even require pins and/or plates to hold the bones together. Certain fractures may require traction with pulleys and weights until the bone has grown together. An Orthopedic specialist should be on your case if you have a fracture that needs treatment.

After a fracture has been "set", you need to be aware of extremity swelling, redness, coldness, numbness, or discoloration and notify your nurse or physician as soon as possible if these symptoms occur. There is also a chance of blood clots due to either the surgery or your immobility related to the fracture. Therapy may be a necessary part of your recovery and should assist with your daily activities during this new condition. The therapy may be in-patient or out-patient, but it will depend on your level of functionality and what your insurance will cover.

After a cast or immobilizing systems are removed, the injured bone has been held in a "fixed" position for usually several weeks. Make sure that you are offered therapy to regain your strength back. I once knew of an 86 year old woman that had fractured her arm and had a cast on for 6 weeks. The physician took the cast off in his office and sent her home. She could not even move her arm as it was weak and "stiff". Be proactive and make sure that you are getting all of the treatment that is necessary for a full recovery.

Preventative Measures

If you have conditions like osteoporosis, follow up with strengthen exercises to increase bone density and take recommended medications as prescribed. Make sure to consume adequate amounts of vitamins and minerals for strong bones.

You can reduce your risk for fractures by wearing your seat belt while in automobiles, along with getting necessary screening for conditions like osteoporosis. If you are at risk for falls, make sure to utilize necessary assistive devices such a walker or cane while walking. Wear protective gear when participating in sports or high risk activities to reduce your risk for fractures.

Cancer

New cells are developing constantly in your body, but sometimes "something" goes wrong. A diagnosis of cancer means that there has been uncontrolled growth of certain cells in your body. Cancer could mean that there is a tumor somewhere in your body or it could be in your blood depending on what type of cancer you have.

Cancer is often "staged" or "graded" by the size and whether it has spread to other places. Those with a higher stage of cancer are the ones that usually need the most aggressive forms of treatments.

Cancer cells can spread, and this is called metastases. Because of so many variables and types of cancer, the treatment plan is developed on an individualized basis and should be implemented by a team of doctors including: your primary care physician, hematologist/oncologist, radiologist and possibly a surgeon. Your primary physician should be overseeing your general well being while the surgeon would be the one to remove the tumor if necessary. The hematologist/oncologist is the one that handles the treatment plan and the radiologist will oversee any necessary radiological treatments or diagnostic testing.

I have worked on an Oncology Unit for several years and have taken care of many cancer patients. Not that long ago, the diagnosis of cancer and death seemed to go hand and hand, but with advances in research, this is a condition that can be beat.

Today, the doctors are going to use treatment plans that have been based on "best practice results". The research has shown if the patient has cancer type "A" and "B" then there is a high success rate if they use treatment "C".

Here is an example:
"Breast cancer" = (A), and it has
"Metastasized to the bone" = (B), then they will use
"Fluorouracil" = (C), as the chemotherapy drug.

A+B=C in this instance.

I have taken something that is very complex because of the number of variables, but I want you to understand the concept of a "pathway". A+B=C was used above, but your condition might have more variables in the equation and look more like A+B+J+M= C & D as recommended treatments. You want to make sure that your treatment plan is following one of these pathways, and that you are receiving the best known treatment for your type and stage of cancer, but it should be customized for your situation.

Cancer develops over years and has usually been in your body for a long time before it is diagnosed. Most cancers when diagnosed do not require emergency treatment to save your life, so make sure that you feel comfortable with your diagnosis, your physicians, and your treatment plan. Remember this did not develop overnight, so slow down and take a deep breath. If you would like a second opinion, please do not hesitate to get one, as you need to trust those that are taking care of you. You need to ask your physician how many cases like yours he has treated, and of course, do research on the physician (see the chapter on finding the best physicians).

When my husband John was 25 years old, he had been having some minor symptoms which included; a mild dizziness and nausea when he was playing basketball, but he just felt he was a "little out of shape". He would sit down on the bench, and the symptoms would go away, so he ignored the symptoms as a lot of people do. Then one day he had the symptoms while sitting at his desk at work. He could not ignore the symptoms anymore.

We started out that day on what was going to be a 3 month journey. The physician ordered the standard blood tests, but everything came back "normal". We went from one test to another with no diagnosis. When days and months go by, you almost get to the point that you wish they would give you a positive diagnosis, just so they could fix it.

Life went on, and one day as we were just pulling into a parking lot, he said to me "what is that smell?" Of course I did not smell anything, but he said it smelled like a bottle of ammonia under his nose. It was at this point, the physician decided to do a CT of the brain. He went in for the test on a Friday night after work, but when he came home, he said that he would need to go back the next morning because there was something wrong with the machine.

The next day, our son and I went along for the ride to the hospital, only to find our physician and the neurosurgeon waiting there to see us. They told us that John had a tumor the size of a tennis ball in his brain. They believed that it was benign (non-cancerous) because of the size, but they could not make the final diagnosis until they removed it. Cancerous tumors tend to grow at a faster rate than benign tumors, and his brain probably would not have accommodated a tumor of that size if it had been fast growing.

There are a couple of things that I must share from this experience. First, it is true when they say that we only remember so much during a traumatic time like this. To this day, I know that our son was not in the room when the doctors told us about John's condition, but I do not remember who I gave the baby to. I am guessing it was some nurse, but that was erased from my memory. It was just too much information for my brain to handle at that time. It is just one more reason to make sure that you have someone with you when you visit the doctor. Have the physician write things down if necessary, so later when you are ready to consider your options you have something other than your "memory" to rely on.

Secondly, they wanted to put my husband in the hospital that day and do surgery immediately. Remember, it has taken years to develop this tumor and you need to make sure that you are making the right decisions. We left the hospital that day because we needed time to get a second opinion. At that point in time, we would have gone wherever we needed to go, and see whatever doctor was best qualified to perform the surgery.

We went to see the head neurologist at Henry Ford Hospital which was about 45 minutes away from us. We knew that they had a wonderful reputation for their neurology department, so there was no question about where we would go for a second opinion.

He looked at John's CT, performed an assessment, and asked about the treatment plan. After listening to what we had to say, it would have been very easy for him to tell us to come there for surgery, but he didn't. He told us that they had been trying for years to get the surgeon from our local hospital on their staff, and that he was one of the top surgeons in the state for this type of surgery.

The local hospital had also just built a new neuro-intensive care unit to this surgeon's specifications. We had a great surgeon and the hospital that could accommodate John's condition. We did our research and in the end, felt very comfortable with our decision. I know that the surgeon was not "happy" the day we left the hospital for a second opinion as he knew the severity of the diagnosis, but remember you are also on the "team", and need to have an active say in what is going to happen to your body. You need to understand the risks or consequences if the treatment is delayed, but also know that you can find peace from obtaining a second opinion.

The symptoms of cancer vary greatly with the location and type of cancer. It is important to report any abnormal symptoms to your physician, but many cancerous tumors are found by accident. A patient was admitted to the hospital for appendicitis, after they performed the diagnostic test, they informed him that he also had a large tumor on his kidney as well as a ruptured appendix. This scenario can complicate treatment plans, and physicians can have different treatment approaches to cases like this.

They removed the appendix, but left the tumor intact. They wanted the patient to "heal" a little before they removed the tumor on the kidney. The appendix had ruptured and if the tumor was removed at the same time, the patient could have been at a greater risk for infection and complications. This was a wise decision made by this physician, but the tumor could have gone undetected until advanced stages, if the diagnostic test had not been performed. All treatment methods tend to be most effective with early detection.

Diagnostic Tests

If you have a diagnosis of cancer, you probably have already gone through or will have some of these diagnostic tests:

     CT (Computed Tomography) Scan
     MRI (Magnetic Resonance Imaging)
     Bone Scan
     PET (Positron Emission Tomography) Scan
     X-Rays
     Ultra Sound
     Blood samples which should include cancer markers.

Genetic testing is optional and usually is not covered by insurances. Until they refine some of the genetic testing, you truly need to understand what the test is telling you. Some positive results could mean that you have a 50 percent chance of developing cancer by the time you are 80 years old. Positive results can create anxiety and undue fear which puts you at a greater risk for developing cancer in the long run. Make sure you understand the ramifications of genetic testing and what you plan on doing with the results.

Treatments

Chemotherapy is a term generally used to describe the treatments used to kill cancer cells directly. You may also hear them referred to as "anti-cancer" drugs. Some medications used in cancer treatment, do not kill the cancer cells directly, but make it difficult for them to thrive in your body. Tamoxifen is a drug, which is a "hormone modifier", because it interferes with estrogen by occupying the receptors in your body. If the estrogen does not have a receptor to "connect" to, then the estrogen levels go down, which reduces the activity of the estrogen-related tumors. There are over 100 different drugs used to treat cancer, and more are developed all the time.

The cancer drugs can be used to control your tumor's growth, to shrink the tumor prior to surgery, to relieve symptoms, to kill minute cancer cells left behind after surgery, or to cure your cancer. Each patient's regiment will vary depending on the location, size, metastasis, and other patient variables. A great resource for Chemotherapy treatment can be found at http://www.chemocare.com/.

If you are undergoing conventional treatments for cancer, you most likely will have some side effects. These side effects could be as mild as a dry mouth, or serve as a life threatening blood clot. You need to know what the risks are and what you could expect from your treatment regiment. Understanding the possible complication can let you know when you should call your doctor.

Chemotherapy can affect everyone differently, so just because your mother had itching with her Chemo treatments, does not mean that you will have the same experience. Communication with your physician of any new symptoms is necessary so they can assess for any possible treatment modifications. Nausea and vomiting are very common with chemotherapy drugs, but we have some wonderful medications that also counteract these symptoms. A website that offers detailed information about Chemotherapy side effects is located at http://www.chemocare.com/managing/.

Clinical Trials

Cancer patients also may seek Clinical Trials for their treatment, but it necessary that you fully understand what a Clinical Trial actually is. Research is usually conducted in the trails to test the effectiveness of new medical treatments. Various types of clinical trials are conducted at facilities all over the world and can have wonderful results, as new treatments are granted approval for widespread use.

Some studies use a preventative approach, where patients are provided treatments that could lower their risk for cancer, or to prevent a recurrence. Screening trials are conducted with the intent of finding cancer prior to the development of any symptoms, while diagnostic trails are conducted with the goal of identifying cancer more accurately.

When a patient has cancer, the treatment trials can be conducted to obtain more information for a selected treatment. The evaluation of new vaccines, drugs, surgeries or radiation therapy can provide best practice initiatives, which could direct future treatment plans. Patients that participate in clinical trials can be provided access to new approaches or treatments. Those that participate in these research studies, can also receive regular medical attention, and may be the first to find success with new initiatives or treatments. Some patients may even find it therapeutic to participate in a clinical trial that could help others in the future.

Clinical trails can also show if treatments are not effective, or if they cause harm. The downside to research is that the treatment methods are generally not proven treatments. Just because they are "new" treatments or methods, does not mean that the standard approaches would not work for you just as well, or even better.

New treatments can also render unexpected results or side

effects, which could be worse than if you had been given the standard treatments. If you decide to participate in a clinical trail, you may not have a choice in the different regiments being studied. Payment of the treatment may not be covered by your insurance, and you may be required to frequent the doctor more often.

There are many people that have gone through clinical trails, for several different conditions, but you need to make sure that it is right for you. Research is consistently being conducted at most major Universities and hospitals, so research the facility as well as the study to make sure it is something you are interested in, and fully understand the risks associated with your participation in a clinical trial prior your acceptance.

Websites on Clinical Trials for Cancer

http://www.cancer.gov/CLINICALTRIALS
http://www.cancertrialshelp.org/
http://www.cancerguide.org/internet_trials.html
http://www.cancercenter.com/about-us.cfm

Reverse Isolation

Another common reason you might find yourself at the hospital if you have cancer is because of low blood counts. The chemotherapy is killing the cancer cells, but in the process, it is also killing the good cells that help keep us healthy. Your oncologist should be monitoring you blood levels and if you have symptoms of extreme weakness, fatigue, or a general ill feeling, you need to notify your physician immediately.

If you are in the hospital with low white cell counts, you may be in what the hospital calls "reverse isolation". It is not that you are necessarily contagious, but the concern is that you are at greater risk for developing infections. Your physician does not want you exposed to the other sick patients in the hospital. Your ability to fight off infection is greatly reduced, and even a mild infection could cost you your life.

While at home, patients that are receiving treatment for their cancer should take their temperature a couple times a day, and notify their physician if it is over 100.5 degrees F. There are a few things that they will also need to avoid if they have a low white cell count:

- Fresh fruits or vegetables
- Raw meats or fish
- Natural cheeses
- Raw eggs
- Frozen or dried fruits
- Anything that may carry bacteria

You will not be allowed to have fresh flowers or plants at most hospitals if you are in "reverse isolation". Family and friends will need to protect you, and that will require them to stay at home, if they are sick. I cannot stress enough how important hand washing is for disease prevention. Not only for the patient, but for all those that enter the room.

Since you know that the chemotherapy is putting you at risk, even if you do not have extremely low blood counts, you still should avoid large crowds, to decrease your exposure to infectious diseases. You need to discuss any immunization with your physician prior to administration and should avoid anyone who has had an immunization in the last 2 weeks. It is necessary to have a preventative mind set in order to come out of the hospital alive if you have cancer and neutropenia (low white cell count).

Holistic Treatment

Cancer treatments are big business for many drug companies, hospitals and physicians. My friend recently diagnosed with cancer was told that her treatment with Chemo would cost around $73,000. She had insurance, but would still have to pay out of pocket several thousand dollars. Because of the cost and undesirable side effects, patients may seek alternative treatment options.

There can be a sense of your health being out of control when you are diagnosed with cancer, and alternative treatments may give you back some of that "control" over your health. There are many alternative cancer treatments out there that are beneficial to your health, while others are unproven and dangerous. Distinguishing between the safe and the unsafe is probably the biggest challenge of alternative medicine.

Today there is no guaranteed "cure" for cancer, but research over the years, whether with holistic or conventional treatments, has provided the cancer patient with new treatment options. The holistic or alternative treatments tend to focus on "natural" alternatives, which alter what you consume or do not consume. The simple concept that many tumors "feed" on sugar, means if your consumption of sugar is decreased or regulated, the cancer could be altered. There are many things that a cancer patient can do, even if they select conventional methods of treatments. Taking a preventative approach should be the first action that you take.

My mother had cancer 25 years ago and is alive today in wonderful health, but I have taken care of some patients that were not so fortunate. Today, my sister has also been diagnosed with cancer and she is seeking a combination of conventional and holistic treatments. The treatment selection can have a direct impact on our survival rate.

So often it is not the cancer that patients die from, it is the results of the treatment and the way our bodies respond. Most physicians cannot tell you about holistic treatment methods as this would be out of their scope of practice, but what I want you to know is, there are many people in this world that have lived with a cancer diagnosis for many, many years and never went through traditional medical treatments. Alternative treatments are aimed at attacking the cancer, returning your body to its natural cancer fighting state, and then focusing on maintaining a remission status.

There are facilities all over the world, as well as those in individual practice, which focus on holistic cancer treatments. You need to find the right treatment for you, and do it soon. I know so many patients that try conventional treatment methods, and when all else fails, they reach for holistic treatments. Because the holistic treatments often focuses on your own body "fighting" the cancer off, it is in your best interest if you seek this method, while your body is still strong. If you wait until the conventional doctors tell you they can do nothing else for you, it may also be too late for holistic treatments to be successful as well.

One critical part of your conventional or holistic treatment is to monitor your progress. Adjustments may be necessary if you take Chemo drugs, and the same is true for alternative treatments. You need a physician that is going to monitor your "whole being", and make the necessary adjustments if you are not responding to the treatment.

Holistic treatments extend beyond natural supplements. Some treatments considered as alternative methods for cancer are immunotherapy, photodynamic, hyperthermia, detoxification, and oxygenation, to name a few. No matter what type of treatment you select, you need to do your research, and make sure it is right for you.

There are even some natural or holistic treatments that have been approved in other countries that show great promise, but may not be offered here in the states. Many celebrities have gone to other countries for alternative treatments and have successfully won their cancer battle. For a list of some of the alternative treatments used successfully in other countries, see:

http://www.alternative-cancer.net/78_alternatives.htm.

The integration of the holistic and conventional worlds in cancer treatments may be one of the biggest innovations that come to fruition in the 21st century. I want to offer you hope, but you also need to take and active part in your treatment by making informed decisions.

Here are a few additional links to alternative treatments:

http://www.sunridgemedical.com/
http://cancertutor.com/

Spirituality and Support for Cancer patients

Cancer not only affects the patient, but also the immediate family and extended family. Often there is a loss of a job with the diagnosis, or the difficulty of trying to complete a job while going through treatment. Life does not stand still just because you have a diagnosis of cancer. The children still need to go to school, dinner needs to be fixed and the lawn needs to be mowed. Learning to balance all of life's activities along with your new diagnosis will benefit your health in the long run.

You need to keep your stress level down, as high stress releases hormones that can cause the cancer to grow. Seek stress reduction classes; meditate on scripture, exercise or whatever helps you relieve stress. As a child of a parent with cancer, I can tell you that your children are afraid of loosing you, to a disease they do not understand. Educate them because the more you know about something, the less there is to be afraid of.

One of the most difficult situations can come from your spouse. You need open communication about their thoughts and feelings as you battle this disease together. Our pastor has a saying that difficult situations are either going to make you bitter or they will make you better. Focusing on your healing is a great way to "get better", but it can be a process.

It is very common for the patient and the family to go through the grieving process with a cancer diagnosis. When the patient is first diagnosed, there can be a sense of "shock" or disbelief. Many patients report that they just feel "numb" to the whole situation. After the initial shock, the patient or family may find themselves in denial. "This cannot be happening to me", it just is not real. Hopefully the patient can move through this stage, as treatments will often be delayed if the patient or family stays in this stage too long.

I knew of a family that had been told that their Mother was

dying, and would probably not make it out of the hospital alive. The husband was in denial and went out the next day and bought tickets for a cruise for him and his wife. Their daughter was very upset with her father, but she did not understand that he was still in the denial phase. Sometimes it is hard for the patient and the family members when they are progressing through these stages at different speeds.

Those with cancer usually experience a time of anger. They are faced with losing their loved ones, and their life has just been turned upside down. The "Why me", question usually is verbalized at this stage. Family members can also go through a time of anger, and the patient needs to understand this, and help them through it.

Bargaining is also a stage where the patient or family reaches out to God and expects that they can be healed if they do "something" for God. Your faith can have such an impact on your outlook which can also affect your disease process. Healing can occur with any disease, and God can have a direct impact on that, but bargaining is driven by our human nature. When faced with reality, there is a good possibility that the patient and family will experience some form of depression as they come to the place of understanding the reality of their condition, or that their bargaining has not been effective.

They may be sad, but also may still feel angry "inside". It is only when the patient and family members reach the acceptance stage that spiritual, physical and mental healing can truly begin. This is not to say that the patient will not experience some form of these stages again, as their condition wavers. Relapses or changes in the patient's condition can cause a regression in the process, and with cancer, you may never know what one day will bring.

A great support system needs to be in place for optimal healing to occur. If those closest to you are not in a condition to support you during this time, then you need to seek outside sources. You need to have someone that understands your ups and downs, and all your thoughts and feelings. There are cancer support groups, but they can also pose difficult situations when a member does not survive their disease. You need people that will lift you up, and be concerned not only for your physical well being, but the mental and spiritual aspects as well. Here are a couple of websites that might be able to help you find a support group in your community.

http://www.cancerhopenetwork.org.
http://www.gildasclub.org/

You can also look for support from your local church family. Even though they might not have "cancer support" groups, they are a great source of support that can be there for you as you are traveling down this cancer road. They also can offer the spiritual aspect of healing, that other groups may not be able to offer. Churches are filled with other people that have gone through difficult situations like your, so reach out and find your optimal support group.

Encourage your spouse and family to join you in support groups, which could assist them during this difficult time. Be understanding of their feelings as their world has also just been turned upside down too. Financial difficulties can also occur when someone is diagnosed with cancer, as this can put a financial strain on the other spouse. There are so many things that change once someone is diagnosed with cancer.

When a child is the one with cancer, it can be a very difficult time for the parents. You need to be united for your child's sake. In tough situations like this, you will either become stronger, or it could break you apart as a couple. Stay strong for you child, as they need to know that they can count on your support.

The life saving treatments can be very expensive, so if you are unable to pay, make sure that you tell your doctor. Many pharmaceutical companies offer assistance if you qualify but you will never know unless you ask. Even if you have insurance, the amount that you will end up paying could be astounding. Make sure to ask about the different treatment options, to avoid financial stress later.

What did you say?

So often those around us may not know what to say, and because of that, bizarre things can come out of their mouths, so just expect it. When my mother had cancer she had a lady tell her "if you can't be cured, you know it is just better to be with the Lord in heaven". My mother had 3 children still at home ages 7, 10 and 20, and she needed every bit of hope she could be given. Although this lady may have had good intentions, it came out all wrong. Sometimes it is better to just say nothing at all if you do not have something kind to say.

If you are trying to encourage those diagnosed with cancer, be sensitive to them by asking how they are doing, or what you can do for them. As simple as it sounds, taking in a meal or offering to pick up the children, may be just what the doctor ordered.

Your attitude towards your condition plays such a part in your recovery, so you need to surround yourself with encouraging people. My mother has always said that there are "life giving people and life draining people", so make careful considerations when selecting your support group.

Cellulitis

This condition is an infection of the skin caused by streptococcal or staphylococcal bacteria that has entered through a break in the skin. Some cases can develop without a break in the skin, but those most at risk for non-wound cellulitis usually have a compromised immune system or diabetes.

Signs and Symptoms

Infection is usually visible on the outer layer of the skin, but can spread to the deeper layers. Most cases are found on the lower extremities, but can occur anywhere. Symptoms can include redness, tenderness, pain and swelling of the affected area. We will see a high fever in some cases, but usually only if the condition has spread.

Treatment

Infections of the face need prompt attention as it could lead to a serious eye infection. If it is on your face, there is also a possibility of it spreading to your brain, causing meningitis. It is important to seek immediate medical attention for cellulitis, because if left untreated, it can lead to sepsis, which could even cause death.

It is not usually a serious condition, but there is a rare type of Cellulitis, commonly referred to as the "flesh eating bacteria". This type should be treated immediately to prevent the tissue from dying as it too can be a life threatening situation.

Blood cultures should be collected before antibiotics are administrated, and depending on the severity of the case, you may be able to take oral antibiotics or IV antibiotics may be required. The physician should draw a line around the affect area to monitor the redness, as this will help assess the status of the infection. The goal would be for the infection or red area to get smaller, but if it starts to go beyond the lines, makes sure to tell your nurse or physician as soon as possible as you may need a different type of treatment. If you are on bed rest or your Cellulitis is on your lower extremities, you may be at risk for blood clots, so anticoagulants may be administered as a preventative measure in this case. You may also be given medication for associated pain or inflammation.

Preventative measures

Keep all cuts covered with a bandage to decrease your exposure to bacteria. Monitor your skin if you have ulcers, eczema, psoriasis or fungal infections which can put you at risk for developing cellulitis. Keep your skin clean and check for cracks or wounds on your skin frequently. If you have a skin infection, make sure to seek treatment, and follow the regiment as prescribed. Changes in wounds need to be addressed by a physician.

Closed Head Injury

A closed head injury can be caused by everything from a car accident to just falling and hitting your head. In cases where injury to the brain has occurred, there is a risk for brain swelling to develop. Just like when you sprain your ankle and it swells, the brain can also respond with swelling when injured. The difference between your ankle injury and your brain injury is that the brain is enclosed by the skull which does not accommodate extreme swelling, and could interfere with brain function. If the brain is injured, the swelling needs to be monitored through several methods.

Signs and Symptoms

Confusion, headache, dizziness, nausea and vomiting are all symptoms of a closed head injury. The doctors and nurses will be assessing the patient frequently for any changes in mental status or physical mobility, and if the patient opens his eyes on his own. The pupils will also be assessed and noted on the size and reaction to light. The patient will also be asked to move extremities and this test should be repeated frequently based on the patient's condition and response. Closed head injuries can have symptoms that occur on just one side of the body, or on both. Loss of consciousness is not a good sign for any closed head injury patient. If you know that a patient has hit their head, it could be very helpful in evaluating the condition or assist with the prompt ordering of diagnostic tests.

I took care of a patient that had a closed head injury that experienced a delay in treatment. He had made some changes in the recommended dose of his anti-seizure medication, without any obvious symptoms. One day he went to take a shower, and locked the door behind him. The patient ended up having a seizure while in the shower, and he fell, and hit his head. Much time elapsed before someone realized that he had been in the bathroom for a long time, and then the door was locked which did not allow for easy access by the children. An ambulance was finally called, and the patient was still unconscious when he arrived at the hospital. Precious time had elapsed, that could have altered this patient's outcome.

I wish that I could give this story a happy ending, but the months that I knew this patient, he did not regain consciousness. There was some brain activity, but he was not a functioning individual because of his closed head injury.

Treatment

Closed head injuries can be classified as mild to severe and with this wide range also comes a wide range of treatments. You could have a mild concussion which does not always require hospitalization, or you could have a condition that the patient has lost consciousness for a brief time, or is even in a coma. In severe cases, drugs are often used to help regulate intracranial pressure, but your condition may also require the physician to insert a device to monitor the pressure level in the brain. Because the brain regulates body function, no matter what the device reading is, if there are symptoms such as respiratory distress, they need to be addressed. For severe closed head injuries, the patient will probably be in the intensive care unit due to the need for one on one assessment and close monitoring.

Depending on the injury, surgery may also be required to relieve the pressure or to repair a blood vessel. Anytime surgery is required, there is the risk for infection, and the brain is really not any place that we want an infection to develop. Usually when the patient requires surgery, the benefits outweigh the risk associated with the surgery. Still you need to make sure that your surgeon is one that can handle your condition.

An unconscious patient will often have multiple IV's, tubes and wires to help monitor their condition or sustain their life. Those unaccustomed to this scenario could be overwhelmed when seeing the patient for the first time. When you have a loved one with severe injuries, you do not always think clearly, so be prepared, and write any questions you have in a notebook. Most physicians are readily available to the patients in the ICU, so do not be afraid to ask for the physician to be contacted if you need information about their condition or treatment.

After my husband's brain surgery, the surgeon said that the tumor was benign, but we would have to watch for meningitis, since they had opened the brain up. When John became conscious, he didn't complain about his head, he complained about his neck. I knew that neck pain was a symptom of meningitis, so I asked that the physician be contacted. As it turned out, the pain in John's neck was due to the position they had him in for surgery. His head was literally put in a vise, which held his head off the table and to one side for many hours. We must remember that we (even the family) are part of the healthcare team. Doctors and Nurses are in the "service" business and they should not mind if someone on "their team" wants to talk to them. If that is a problem for your physician, you need to evaluate your relationship and if this is a good situation for you or the patient.

Prevention

Prevention is the best recommendation for closed head injuries. If you are unsteady on your feet, make sure to remove clutter on the floor, and use assistive devices if necessary. Make sure you have proper lighting to avoiding falls that could result in a head injury, and always wear seat belts while in automobiles incase of an accident.

There are around 570,000 patients each year with closed head injuries and it is the leading cause of death in children and adults less than 46 years of age. Depending on the severity of the condition, you could expect just an ER visit or a short hospital stay. There is also the chance of the recovery taking months or even requiring a life spent in a long term nursing facility. A closed head injury can be very devastating and may require many days of rehabilitation depending on the severity of the injury. It all depends on the level of injury and how the patient responds to the treatment.

There is a high probability of death associated with closed head injuries as approximately 100,000 people will not survive their injury each year. Evaluation is the best thing you can do when a head injury has occurred. The actress Natasha Richardson recently hit her head while skiing, but felt she was ok, and denied treatment. She later died of her closed head injury, so it is important to not dismiss common symptoms of headache, confusion, dizziness, nausea and vomiting. Other subtle symptoms are insomnia, irritability, trouble concentrating, and intolerance to bright lights or loud noises. If a head injury has occurred, seek treatment immediately to optimize your treatment and recovery.

Chronic Obstructive Pulmonary Disease (COPD)

Patients with COPD, a potentially fatal lung disease, have been diagnosed with Asthma, Chronic Bronchitis, Chronic Obstructive Bronchitis or Emphysema. COPD is a very common disorder in the United States and is associated greatly with smoking, exposure to highly polluted areas, or a family history of respiratory diseases.

In this condition the patient's airways become narrow, which causes a decreased flow of air to and from the lungs. The body's inflammatory response can also lead to destruction of the lung tissues. The obstruction of the airflow usually develops over time, reducing the amount of air you can exhale.

COPD is the fourth leading cause of death in the United States and can cause an extreme amount of suffering. Anytime a patient has difficulty breathing it can be a scary situation, not only for the patient, but for those around them. With COPD, the patient can experience acute exacerbations, usually brought on by infections or air pollution. It is estimated that $42 billion is spent on issues related to COPD treatments or loss of productivity every year.

Signs and Symptoms

The most common symptom of this condition is difficulty in breathing during exertion. It can even get to the point were you can experience this difficulty just while sitting still. COPD patients can develop a chronic productive cough or a wheezing that occurs when breathing, discoloration of the skin, or even heart failure. If you are experiencing anorexia or weight loss with COPD, your health could be declining.

Treatment

When you arrive at the hospital with COPD symptoms, pulmonary function test and X-rays should be done for evaluation of the disease. Occasionally, a CT may also be performed of the chest for further evaluation.

The goal for COPD treatment is to lessen the airflow restriction, prevent other complications and improve your quality of life. If you have COPD, treatment with bronchodilators, oxygen, steroids and antibiotics could all be ordered. In severe cases, mechanical ventilation may be required, and the patient will be monitored closely in the ICU. In rare cases, surgery may also be performed to remove sections of the diseased lung.

There are certain breathing techniques that can help strengthen the muscles and aid in moving secretions. Pulmonary rehabilitation is also a great resource that can assist with these techniques and can help to gain control of the disease. Ask your physician if you are a candidate for a program like this if it is not automatically offered to you.

Prevention

On a positive note, this condition can be prevented in most cases. Prevention methods include limiting air pollutant exposure, quit smoking, or do not smoke to begin with. Stay healthy and wash your hands frequently to try to avoid respiratory infections if you have been diagnosed with COPD. Receiving the Pneumonia or Flu vaccines could be beneficial if your physician approves of them for your condition, but receiving the vaccine does not guarantee you will not develop the condition. The foremost thing you can do for yourself is quit smoking, if you have not already. Continually filling the lungs with pollutants found in cigarettes can cause COPD or exacerbate the condition once it has developed. Damage to your lungs cannot usually be reversed, so the symptoms are also treated in hopes of reducing the risk for further damage.

Living with COPD can alter your lifestyle as you may have to give up activities that you used to do. A good support system needs to be in place for those living with this condition. Seek help from your family and friends, or those that have gone through this before. If you are feeling depressed about your condition, you may benefit from counseling, and ask your physician if he has any information that would help you to cope with your disease. For those having trouble quitting smoking, talk with your physician about medication options that may assist with this task.

Diabetes

This is a general term used to describe several different conditions that fall under this diagnosis. Gestational Diabetes occurs in pregnant women, which is usually discovered during a routine doctor's office visit, and often resolves after the pregnancy ends. There is some research that indicates that having Gestational Diabetes can put the individual at a higher risk for developing Type 2 Diabetes later on in life.

Type 1 Diabetes is caused when your body's immune system basically turns against the insulin producing cells as though they were foreign invaders. It is for this reason that people with Type 1 diabetes are required to take insulin injections. We see an increased risk for kidney and heart disease, and blindness in these patients as well. This condition usually is discovered in childhood and is often called juvenile diabetes, but can develop in adults as well.

Type 2 Diabetes is most commonly found in the adult population and reports estimate that nearly 20 million people are affected with this disease and another 45 million individuals are in a pre-diabetic state. With type 2, there is a problem with the way your body metabolizes glucose for energy. Those with type 2 may produce insulin, but it may not be enough or is not used properly by the body. With the lack of insulin, the glucose that is consumed in the body is not utilized, and results in a high amount of glucose in the blood stream. This can be somewhat controlled through diet and exercise, but this condition can also be life-threatening. The doctors would like to see a fasting glucose level (no food overnight) in the 70-100 range. If you are over 45, your glucose levels should be evaluated annually as prevention is always the best method.

Diabetes Signs and Symptoms

If you are experiencing symptoms such as increased thirst, increased urination, weight loss, numbness, or have the need to eat an abnormal amount of food, you should be seen a physician. Diabetes is a very serious condition and has been associated with or may even be the cause of heart disease, peripheral vascular disease, stroke, high blood pressure, cancer, and obesity.

Treatment

If you are in the hospital with a new diagnosis of diabetes, they will determine what type, so the proper treatment and education can be provided. In order to effectively manage this condition there will need to be a change in your life style. Education topics will include diet modifications, exercise, medication administration, how to monitor your blood sugar levels and recognize abnormal symptoms. There are many topics that need to be covered thoroughly if you are diabetic, but one key component associated with insulin injection is to rotate the sites to avoid a condition called lipodystrophy, which can cause damage to the tissue. Most physicians can recommend educational classes on this topic, but inquire if the information is not automatically provided.

Low Blood Sugar Levels

Hypoglycemia is when your blood sugar gets too low and you may experience nervousness, sweating, weakness, fatigue, palpitations, tremors, shaking, blurred vision, headache, confusion or seizures. For this condition, it is very important that you get some form of glucose, like fruit juice, soda, graham crackers or sugar cubes right away. It will be beneficial for you to consume a meal as the symptoms get better to obtain some protein and carbohydrates as well.

Be proactive in your treatment and make informed decisions. It is very easy for a physician to prescribe a medication because they think it is easier for you to take a pill than to modify a lifestyle. There are risk associated with the medications used to treat diabetes so research all medications you are prescribed.

In some combinations, drugs can have devastating results. Because we all metabolize (break things down so our body can use it) substances we consume differently, each individual can have various reactions. For example, if my mother takes a Benadryl (Antihistamine) she would sleep for the next day. It just has that affect on her, but I could take a Benadryl and could go work a midnight shift without any problems. Some might say my mother is just experiencing the side effects, but what I am trying to tell you is that medication can affect people differently. Having a complete understanding of your treatment and how the medication affects you is very relevant information for those with diabetes.

High Blood Sugar Levels

Hyperglycemia is when your blood glucose is too high. This can also be caused by illnesses, stress or excess food. We often see an increase in glucose with patients in the hospital. Some signs and symptoms of this condition is nausea, vomiting, thirst, lethargy, increased temperature, flushed skin, dry mouth, irritability, tachycardia, coma and a fruity breath smell. I have seen patients with blood glucose levels at 750 and at 45 with very little symptoms, but in these cases, the patients can "crash" very fast. Diabetics need to listen to their body and if something seems out of the ordinary, make sure the blood glucose levels are evaluated.

Your family members also need to know the signs and symptoms of abnormal glucose levels, and how to treat the condition. To help regulate your disease you may need to see an endocrinologist who specializes in treating diabetes. In some cases there are patients that even have insulin pumps implanted in their abdomen to help regulate their glucose levels.

Most diabetic patients require a visit to the hospital because of complications of their disease, and it is usually because their glucose levels are either too high or too low. Hospital treatment will entail regulating the glucose levels and determining the causation. The way your body responds to the treatment will determine the number of days you will stay in the hospital.

Other Complications

Although the list of complications associated with Diabetes is long, there are a few that are seen frequently at the hospital. The excess glucose in your blood can injure the small capillaries that feed your nerves. This produces a neuropathy which can cause pain, burning, numbness or tingling, which generally starts in the toes or fingers. Wounds and diabetics just seem to go hand and hand. Because patients often experience neuropathy or poor blood flow in their feet, they may have cuts that go undetected until an infection has developed. Patients may also develop gangrene in their extremities, which could even require amputation of the affected digit or limb. The poor healing associated with diabetic patients can render a very slow healing process, which could take months or even years.

Diabetics need to have a thorough evaluation of their feet, on a regular basis, especially if the patient has neuropathy. If they are not able to examine their own feet, someone will need to do this for them. Having a podiatrist trim the toenails can also reduce the risk for injury as well as wearing the proper shoes.

Alternative Treatments

My father who is 70 years old was just diagnosed with this type 2 diabetes a few months ago. First he was faced with the new task of checking his blood sugar levels, and now this is a very big task for my father who does not like the sight of blood. My parents live out of state so I am not involved with their care as much as I would like to be, so my Dad had the nurse show him how to "poke" his finger in the doctor's office and put the blood drop on the glucometer. Sounded easy enough, right? After he told me that he tried 13 times to get the machine to work, I knew there was something wrong. He was missing the key instruction of "how" to put the blood on the strip. He thought you just set it on top of the strip, when actually he needed to put it on the end and let the strip draw it up into the device for the actual results. If you are having difficulty, check with your physician immediately, as it is not suppose to be a difficult task.

The doctor wanted to put my father on oral medications to control his glucose level, but after a little encouragement from me, he chose to change his diet and exercise first. In a couple of months he has lost 30 pounds and his glucose levels have returned to very acceptable levels. This may not be an option for you, but if you can take one less medication a day, it is worth talking to your physician about. There are also natural herbs like Cinnamon that have been associated with increased glucose metabolism that may also be beneficial. Implementing good fats into your diet, reducing non-fiber carbohydrates/starches, and exercise could all be the key to controlling or even totally reversing this condition.

Hepatitis

Hepatitis is a term utilized for several different diseases that causes an inflammation of the liver. Hepatitis A can be acquired through contaminated food or water, while other types of Hepatitis are transmitted through blood or body fluids. Hepatitis can be mild to severe or even life threatening. Most Hepatitis B cases are acute or short term and the body is able to fight the virus off, but sometimes the infection becomes chronic, lasting longer than 6 months. If the liver is damaged beyond repair, it can become hardened, and cirrhosis can develop. Some cases of Hepatitis can also lead to liver cancer.

Signs and Symptoms

The condition is usually diagnosed with a blood test to determine your liver enzymes. The condition can present with symptoms of being jaundice (yellowing of the skin and eyes), a change in mental status or other system failures.

Treatment

Mild cases are usually treated in the office setting, but if severe, the patient may need to be hospitalized. For Hepatitis A, it can take 2 weeks to several months to recover, while others with Hepatitis B may never totally get over the condition. Some key elements in this condition include how to prevent the spread of this disease. There are vaccines now that can protect you from this disease so that would be the best scenario. If you already have this condition, antibiotics may be prescribed. For more details on Hepatitis, see the chapters later in the book on hospital acquired infections.

Prevention

Education on proper handwashing is a key element for prevention of spreading the infection. Family members should avoid contact with infected body fluids. Those with multiple sex partners, homosexual men, drug abusers, babies born to "positive for hepatitis" mothers, and healthcare workers are at greatest risk, so make sure to protect others if you are given this diagnosis.

Hypercholesterolemia (High Cholesterol)

High cholesterol is generally a condition that in and of itself does not usually bring you to the hospital. Cholesterol is not necessarily a "bad" thing, as our body does need it to help with metabolism or to produce certain hormones. The risk occurs because high levels of cholesterol in your blood can deposit in the arteries, leaving you at risk for developing coronary artery disease. High cholesterol can be an inherited factor or caused by certain medications or diseases. A high fat diet is one of the leading causes of this condition, so diet modification is one thing you can control that may prevent this from developing.

Signs and Symptoms

This condition does not usually carry any symptoms by itself, so blood tests are the best indicators to diagnosis elevated levels. Routine screenings should be conducted to keep this within a normal level. Once someone has experienced complications associated with high cholesterol, then treatment and lifestyle modifications should be initiated..

Treatments

There are several drugs on the market, generally referred to as "Statins", which are prescribed to help lower your cholesterol, but understand that it could be possible for you to regulate your cholesterol with a low fat diet and exercise. There are millions of people taking these drugs, and the sad part is, they do not know all the possible side effects.

As a nurse I often have family and friends come to me with medical questions, and I have received more on these drugs and their side effects in the last year, than any other. The family members of patients on the statins were the ones with the questions, as the patients do not always notice any side affects.

Most questions focused on how the drugs affect the patient's memory or mood. At first I looked to my drug guide to make sure I was not missing something, but I did not see these types of symptoms. As I mentioned before, side effects of drugs are found on an individual basis, but these reported symptoms were not listed in the drug guide. After several months of the same questions from various individuals, I researched the topic again, and broadened my scope to find more detailed information.

The neurological effects of these medications can have devastating ramifications not only for the patient, but also for the family members. Study results often depend on who is conducting the research, but it does look like doctors are now starting to report memory loss in their patients that take statin drugs. The memory loss associated with these drugs does not matter if you are 40 or 70 years of age, it just can have this affect. I knew a 48 year old patient that was constantly leaving his keys or cell phone at random locations, which had never been a problem before. For this individual, his cell phone was his life line to his work, and he knew the importance it was to his business.

Another call came from my brother who works with my Father every day. He called and reported that Dad was asking him the same questions three to four times in one hour, and my mother confirmed this along with his irritability. I first questioned his age, because he is getting close to 70, but it just came on so fast. Then I found out that his physician had just doubled the dose of his statin drug a few weeks prior. Bingo! I was almost certain that we had found the culprit to the memory loss.

I wanted to know what the natural or holistic alternatives were to lowering cholesterol, and we found that red rice yeast is often given to reduce high cholesterol and does not have the memory loss side effects. Garlic also helps to keep the blood from clotting, so we have included this into his daily regiment and took him off the statin drugs. I do not recommend you just stop taking your medication, but I do advise you to be aware of the side effects and work with your physician to find out what is best for you. At my father's last doctor's visit, his blood levels were the best they had been in years and his physician was thrilled.

Another friend of mine has been dealing with cholesterol levels well into the 300s for years, and even with the statin drugs found it very difficult to bring this level down. He had been experiencing some of the same memory loss issues, so I told him about the Red Rice Yeast. After a couple of months on the Red Rice Yeast, he returned to his physician for another cholesterol analysis. His cholesterol level was 209, which he had not seen for quite some time and the memory loss improved. His physician recommended that he continue on this holistic regiment. It may not be for everyone, but make informed decisions when it comes to your healthcare decisions.

Mayo Clinic also associates a link between statin use and amyotrophic lateral sclerosis (ALS or Lou Gehrig's disease), which is a very devastating condition. Before taking the statin drugs, you must fully consider the risks, the benefits and the alternatives. Some common side effects of the statin drugs are usually provided with your medication from the pharmacy, but can include digestive problems like nausea, diarrhea or constipation.

The Mayo Clinic lists on their website that patients taking statin drugs may experience muscle pain, and even to the point of it interfering with your daily activities. There is also a serious condition called Rhabdomylosis where the muscles breakdown and send myoglobin into the blood stream, resulting in possible liver damage, kidney failure or even death. This condition can present rather fast as a patient once described to me.

She was going to a University of Michigan football game and as they parked the car, she was symptom free, but by the time she reached the stadium, she could not walk. It is very common for patients on statins to experience pain so if you have any questions, it is better to contact your doctor than to ignore the symptoms, and have irreversible damage to your liver or kidneys. This is truly a condition that it is better to be safe, than sorry that you did not seek medical attention sooner.

Prevention

Prevention will include adopting a healthy life style, which includes a low fat diet and exercise. Unless your physician tells you otherwise, you should aim for 7 percent (or less) of your total calories coming from saturated fat and consuming less than 200 mg of cholesterol per day.

If you are overweight, weight reduction can aid in lowering cholesterol levels. Adding fiber to your diet, which is found in fruits, vegetables and grains, is also a good way to help reduce cholesterol. The National Heart, Lung and Blood institute has come up with some suggestions for your grocery list that might help lower your cholesterol levels. The list can be found at:

http://www.emedicinehealth.com/high_cholesterol/page8_em.htm

Monitoring your cholesterol levels should be reviewed annually. If you are on medication to treat high cholesterol, the levels should be checked more frequently. Most physicians would like to see the cholesterol serums be less than 200 mg/dl, LDL cholesterol between 60-180 mg/dl and HDL cholesterol between 30 to 80 mg/dl. Find out what your levels are and take the necessary steps to maintain an acceptable level. Just make sure that you implement the treatments that are right for you.

High Blood Pressure (Hypertension or HTN)

High Blood Pressure is a condition that affects millions of Americans, but is often called the silent killer. The heart pumps thousands of times just in one day, which is a necessary function for our survival. The blood is pushed through the arteries, and when there is great resistance to this, you can develop what is called hypertension (HTN), or high blood pressure. Many patients will be diagnosed with HTN in the physician's office, or in the hospital setting, but many do not even know that they have this condition.

Hypertension is now on the rise after years of decline and is believed to affect 1 in 4 individuals living in the United States, which correlates to as many as 60 million Americans. Several different conditions that can cause hypertension include vascular, renal, endocrine, and neurological disorders. "White coat syndrome", acute stress, medications and even certain foods like cheese, yeast, beer and wine can all cause the blood pressure to rise. Research studies have also related an increased risk of dying during a heart attack if the patient has high blood pressure, and the percentage of risk goes up, as the blood pressure rises.

Secondary hypertension can be related to pregnancy, birth control pills, alcohol addiction, thyroid dysfunction, tumors, sleep apnea and kidney disease. In some cases, you can remove the "stimulant" and the blood pressure will go down, but in chronic cases, it can be more difficult to control.

Certain factors can also affect your blood pressure. As you age, you have a greater risk of HTN as your arteries get stiffer. If you are an African American, you also tend to have higher blood pressure, and the condition may develop sooner than seen in other races. Those in lower socioeconomic statuses can develop HTN more frequently because they may not have the education on how to prevent the condition. HTN also tends to have a heredity factor, but this could be related to families having the same kind of diets. Men have a greater probability of HTN as does those that are obese. If you have hypertension, you have a greater risk for having a heart attack or stroke.

Signs and Symptoms

There are not clear cut signs and symptoms of high blood pressure, other than the elevated reading. Systolic (the top reading) number of 140 mm Hg or higher, and diastolic (the bottom reading) number of 90 mm Hg or higher, could indicate that you have high blood pressure, but a one time reading of high blood pressure does not necessarily mean that you have chronic hypertension. It is necessary to evaluate the situation with more than one reading and possibly over different days.

If you have a severe headache, faintness, blurred vision, light-headedness, dizziness, nausea, chest pain, weakness or shortness of breath, you need to seek immediate medical attention, as these could all indicate complications associated with high blood pressure.

Treatment

Patients with complications associated with high blood pressure may require hospitalization. It may be necessary to administer intravenous medications, to decrease the patient's blood pressure, depending on what is causing it. Usually this will either need to be done on a cardiac unit or in the ICU as you will need to be monitored very close during this treatment. There is usually a cardiologist consulted and the blood work should be evaluated. Major arteries are usually scanned to determine if there are any blockages that could be causing the high blood pressure.

If you have this diagnosis and there are no major blockages, your physician will often look next at your lifestyle and make recommendations that could have an impact on your blood pressure. A low sodium, low fat diet and restrictions on caffeine and alcohol can have a dramatic affect on your blood pressure. For many this is a very difficult lifestyle change.

If the family is supportive, we find a better compliance with these recommendations. An exercise regiment should also be a part of your daily activities if you have hypertension, but always check with your physician prior to exercise initiation. With the exercise regiment and dietary changes we usually see weight loss, which can also aid in lowering the blood pressure. Your physician can tell you how many calories you should be consuming during your weight reduction and maintenance efforts.

Relaxation techniques such as biofeedback and muscle relaxation techniques can also lower blood pressure. If you have ever had a physician tell you to think about some "far away place" and just relax, he is guiding you through an easy relaxation technique. Classes are often provided in relaxation techniques through local community education or colleges. Check with your physician for recommendations if you want more information on these techniques.

Another lifestyle change includes smoking cessation. Smoking causes the blood vessels to constrict resulting in an increase in the blood pressure. When I think of constricting, I think of a 15 foot Anaconda wrapped around its prey. It usually does not end up in a very good outcome for the prey. The more you smoke the greater your risk for hypertension. Smoking can be a very difficult habit to break, but it is possible, and there are new medications on the market all the time that might work for you, so check with your physician for more information.

Prevention

Maintaining a proper diet, high in fiber, low in fat and sodium can be one way to reduce your risk for HTN. Exercising regularly is also something you can do that will decrease your risk associated with HTN, so contact your physician to provide a personalized regiment for diet and exercise. Know the risk factors that cannot change, such as your age, race, socioeconomic status and gender, and have frequent blood pressure screening by your health care provider to stay on top of this very common condition.

Kidney Stones

If you have ever experienced a kidney stone, I do not have to tell you that it can be a very painful experience. The stones generally consist of salts and minerals in the urine, which forms small stones. There are various sizes of stones, ranging from a fleck of sand to golf-ball size. Even the smallest stone can produce excruciating pain, which could result in a trip to the hospital. The stones can be located in the kidneys, the ureter (tubes between the kidney and bladder), or the bladder, but most symptoms occur when the stone is in the kidney or ureter. It is an abnormal balance in the water, minerals and salts in the urine that can cause stone formation. Dehydration is the most common cause, but also can be a result of medical conditions or a family history of this condition.

Signs and Symptoms

Symptoms can start out mild with general pain in the flank (just above the waist) area, that can also wrap around to the front of your body. Some patients experience extreme pain, blood in the urine and fever. Most patients with kidney stone pain say that they have never experienced anything more painful in their life.

Treatment

Ultra-Sound, X-rays or a CT of the kidneys may be done to identify the stone, but sometimes it can be hard to locate. Expect to be treated with pain medications and IV fluids. Blood work should also be done to establish your calcium levels and see how the kidneys are functioning. Your urine should be "strained" to see if the stone passes. This can be done by either urinating directly through the strainer or by urinating in a container, then pouring the urine through the strainer.

There are some kidney stone cases that will require either lithotripsy (shock waves used to break up the stone), or some form of surgical intervention. If the stone is in the ureter (tube from the kidney to the bladder), the physician may need to perform a surgical procedure where they go up through the bladder and remove the stone. It may be necessary to place a stent in the ureter, to help it stay open, so urine can drain from the kidney to the bladder. After the ureter has healed, the physician will need to go back in and retrieve the stent, usually a few weeks later. Antibiotics may also be prescribed if there is an indication of infection. Most patients are able to pass the kidney stones with vigorous hydration. Once the stone is past or removed, it should be sent to a lab for evaluation which will reveal the composition, and allow for more focused prevention methods.

Prevention

If you have stones that are composed of oxalate or calcium oxalate, you may need to alter your consumption of rhubarb, spinach, chocolate, beets, tea, strawberries, wheat bran, draft beer, soy products or nuts, to name a few.

Vitamin C can also produce oxalate when digested in the body, so check with your physician if you are taking supplements that contain it. Diets high in sugar, sodium and animal protein have also been associated with the development of kidney stones. Some medications may also put you at risk for developing kidney stones and should be evaluated when preventative measures are considered.

Pneumonia

Pneumonia is an infection or inflammatory illness of the lungs. The inflammation can cause the air-filled sacs in the lungs to fill with fluid, which reduces the body's ability to absorb oxygen. This condition can be caused by bacteria, but can also result from the inhalation of food, fluids, dust, smoke or chemicals. Those most vulnerable to this condition include the elderly, individuals that have smoked, have a history of respiratory infections, a weakened immune system, chronic diseases and immobility. Around 3 million individuals in the United States will develop pneumonia each year, and the CDC reports that around 58,000 deaths occur each year, which puts this condition as the sixth leading cause of death.

If you have another condition like heart disease, stroke, seizures, swallowing problems, drug abuse or alcoholism, you are also at a greater risk for developing pneumonia. Once you are exposed to the infective agent, the condition can develop rapidly, and can be difficult for the patient to fight off. Patients in the ICU are also at greater risk for developing pneumonia, due to their health condition, and the treatments that may be necessary to treat them.

Patients in the ICU are often intubated, which assists with respiratory function. Intubation increases the risk not only for pneumonia, but for methicillin-resistant staphylococcus aureus (MRSA) pneumonia, which does not respond to many antibiotics. MRSA is discussed in more detail in the chapters on hospital acquired infections.

Signs and Symptoms

Most patients will have coughing, fever, chills, headache, sputum or a general ill feeling. Sputum may be discolored or blood tinged, and the patient may also report shortness of breath. Some chest pain could develop if the pleura becomes involved. Children can also become lethargic and have a fever, but may not have any specific signs of chest infection.

In elderly patients we may not find common symptoms either, but may find a change in their mental status. This is true for other conditions as well. The elderly population does not always present with the "normal" symptoms for many conditions, they just show up at the emergency room because they are confused, only to find out that they have a bladder infection. Anytime there is a change in mental status, you should really be evaluated by your physician.

Treatments

The diagnosis is usually made after the patient is assessed and chest X-rays are reviewed. If you are coughing up phlegm (sputum), the physician will try to culture it so the best treatment regiment can be administered. Pneumonia is caused by several different organisms, so the treatment can be different from one individual to another. If the pneumonia is caused by bacteria, an antibiotic will usually be prescribed for the condition. There also are antiviral medications that can be administered for viral pneumonia. Antibiotics are generally not prescribed for aspiration pneumonia unless there are other complications.

If they cannot obtain a specimen to culture, then the patient is usually provided a broad spectrum antibiotic. In some cases it is necessary to do a bronchoscopy for an exact diagnosis. You should expect blood work and a possible urine culture to make sure the bacteria has not gone systemic (spread to other areas of the body). Tests may also be performed to rule out tuberculosis, if the condition is suspected, which will require the patient to be in isolation until the test results are complete in two to three days.

Pneumonia can occur in one section of a lung, the whole lung or both lungs. Hospitalized patients will generally be on antibiotics, oxygen and respiratory treatments. The physician should be monitoring the patient's fluid and nutritional intake to make sure they are maintaining adequate nutrition status which can also help fight off the infection. It may be necessary to provide suctioning to the patient, especially those with a tracheostomy or on a ventilator. A pulse oxygen reading should also be evaluated to assess the patient's progression.

Pneumonia is a very treatable condition with all of the antibiotics available today, but if the patient has other medical conditions, the risk for complications increases. The patient should perform coughing and deep breathing exercises at least every couple of hours to help with lung expansion. If the patient's condition allows, there should also be an increase of fluid intake. If the patient is diagnosed with pneumonia, and has been either in the hospital or a long term care facility, there is a possibility that the pneumonia is caused by the MRSA bacteria, and precautions should be taken.

Our daughter had a friend in the hospital for several weeks that she visited almost every day. One day she just happened to mention that her friend did not have a room mate anymore. I immediately considered isolation due to his condition and the risk for infection, but no one at the hospital said anything to her about this condition. Our daughter came down with an upper respiratory infection that required three different antibiotics for her to get over the infection. We did not know for sure if she had developed the same infection as her friend, but you need to fully understand the condition of the person you are visiting in the hospital, and the organisms you could be exposed to. Usually there is a sign on the patient's door that could indicate that the patient is in isolation, so make sure to read the "fine print" before entering the room.

Prevention

If someone is in isolation, you need to know why, and what you need to do to protect yourself. Handwashing is a key preventative, but you may also be required to wear a mask and gown when entering the room for your own protection. The risk of pneumonia is increased by smoking, so to reduce this risk, you need to quit.

There is also a pneumonia vaccine that is recommended for individuals over age 65, or those with chronic health issues, but make sure that your physician feels it would be beneficial for you. The latest research indicates that the vaccine should only be administered once over an individual's life time. Pneumonia can be a life-threatening condition, but eating a proper diet and getting regular exercise can also assist the body in preventing this infection.

Pressure Ulcers

Pressure ulcers can develop in patients in the hospital, long term care facilities, or even at home. They are caused by an injury to the skin that most often occurs due to the patient sitting or lying in one position for too long. Patients that are bedridden or are in wheelchairs have the highest incident rates, but pressure ulcers can develop even in short periods of time. Constant pressure on boney points like the hips, knees and heels can reduce the blood supply to that area, and can cause the tissue to die, but other related causes also need to be considered.

Damage to the skin can occur just by turning the patient from side to side. This condition is called friction. Skin that has been affected by friction is more susceptible to pressure ulcers, so turning a patient carefully can reduce the patient's risk for ulcers related to this condition.

Another cause for pressure ulcer development is when you move in one direction, and your skin moves in another, as this is called shearing. Patients that slide in chairs or beds can stretch or tear the cell walls or small blood vessels, setting up the right conditions for pressure ulcer development. Make sure patients have adequate support to prevent shearing.

Most pressure ulcers can be prevented, but reports from the Journal of American Medical Association (JAMA) site that the incident rates in health care facilities is on the rise, estimating as high as 38 percent in some hospitals. Billions of dollars are spent on pressure ulcer treatments each year, and most ulcers can be prevented. Even though the ulcers can develop outside of the hospital setting, the JAMA estimates that acute care facilities will treat 2.5 million patients in the United States this year for pressure ulcers. It is no small matter when you consider that nearly 60,000 patients will die each year from complications associated with pressure ulcers they have acquired while in the hospital. Even if the pressure ulcer does not take the patient's life, it could be a very long recovery process, as wounds can take weeks or even months to heal.

Symptoms

Pressure ulcers are "staged" or categorized by the severity. In a **Stage I**, the patient's skin around the pressure ulcer is red and does not turn white when you press on the area. The patient may report that the area hurts or even itches. With these early symptoms, the pressure ulcer is just starting to develop. For patients with dark colored skin, it may be difficult to see the reddened area. It may take on more of a blue or purplish cast. Minor signs of pressure ulcers may not truly portray the actual condition as the muscle and tissue below the skin is more susceptible to injury than the visible skin.

Stage II involves the deterioration of the epidermis and/or dermis (the outer layer) layers of the skin. This stage is still considered to be a superficial wound and presents as an abrasion, shallow crater or blister. An open sore can also form when an area of the tissue dies, which puts the patient at greater risk for infection. The skin around the sore may also be irritated and red.

Stage III ulcers develop when an extensive amount of damage has occurred to the tissues located below the skin. These wounds are generally seen as "deep craters" in the patient's subcutaneous tissue. In this stage the wound has not reached the underlying fascia, but is a serious condition for the patient. The patient is also at risk for infection in these open wounds.

Stage IV is the most severe type of pressure ulcer as it involves a great amount of skin loss as well as damage to muscles, bones, tendons and joints. The necrosis or "dead tissue" can extend deep into underlying tissue. These wounds are the most difficult to treat and are the most life threatening.

Complications

Infection from the pressure ulcer can travel into the blood stream and spreads throughout the body causing a condition called Sepsis. In this condition, the infection can cause possible life-threatening shock or organ failure in a short amount of time. The development of sepsis is one of the greatest dangers associated with pressure ulcers.

Cellulitis, which is an infection, can develop in the connective tissue. This is a very painful condition and can lead to life-threatening complications. Bone and joint infections that develop as a result of ulcers, can damage the cartilage, and tissue below the wound in a short period of time. Conditions like Osteomyelitis may go on for years if treatment is not provided. Infections can even lead to bone death which can inhibit movement of the joints and limbs.

Necrotizing fasciitis, commonly known as the flesh-eating bacteria, can destroy the tissue around the muscles, and can cause death within 12-24 hours if not treated. Pain, fever and extensive swelling are early symptoms that require immediate attention. Another condition that requires immediate attention is gangrene.

Notable changes in the tissues suddenly occur within minutes once gangrene develops in pressure ulcers. The toxins produced by the bacteria responsible for gangrene destroys muscle tissue and can result in fatal systemic problems. These conditions often make treating pressure ulcers a challenge, and even life threatening.

Treatments

The best treatment would be for the wound to never happen in the first place, but once a wound has occurred, treatment depends on the stage of the wound and the patient's condition. This can be a slow process on the road to healing as open wounds can be very slow to close. Tissues that have been damaged or destroyed never return to their original condition even if they do heal.

Relieving the pressure of the affected area is a key component for healing to occur. Stage I and II ulcers can usually be treated effectively with conservative measures. Minor, frequent adjustments to position can relive the pressure. For those in a wheelchair, this repositioning should occur about every 15 minutes, while patients in bed should be moved every two hours. This may require assistance for patients that are unconscious or unable to move themselves. Specialty surfaces like mattresses or beds can also be utilized in relieving the pressure points. Some mattresses even provide a constant slow movement of the patient for rotation. These beds are especially nice for patients in the ICU that may have multiple drains or tubes to work around when moving the patient. A nurse or physician will need to request the specialty mattresses, but if you have a loved one in an ICU situation or on bedrest, make sure they have some form of specialty mattress or bed in place.

Wounds should be clean and bandaged, as dressings are used to protect the skin, but are also used to encourage healing. Avoid rubbing the affected area which can cause further damage to the already compromised tissue. There are many different products out on the market designed for wound treatment, so make sure you have someone that specializes in wound care assessing the wound for proper treatment regiment. If gauze dressings are used, it will need to be changed at least once a day. Some of the newer dressings function differently, are see-through and can stay on for several days. It is important to know when the dressing needs to be changed to assure that this process gets done at the proper time.

The Wound VAC is a device that utilizes negative pressure to assist with wound healing. The wound is packed with a foam dressing and then an occlusive dressing is placed on top of the skin. There is a tube that is connected to the dressing and then to a vacuum unit. When the negative pressure is applied, there is an increased blood flow to the wound area. It provides a "closure" to the wound while decreasing the bacterial colonization. Excess fluid is removed and collected in a reservoir attached to the VAC. The VAC is used on patients with Stage III or IV ulcers, and is also indicated for patients with ulcers associated with other medical conditions. Patients with necrotic tissue, osteomyelitis, cancer in the wound, or a fistula may not be able to use a Wound VAC.

Surgery is sometimes required to remove the dead tissue as it can interfere with wound healing. In some cases the dead tissue can be removed by using special dressings that dissolve the dead tissue. These dissolving type dressings are usually left in place for several days at a time. There are also medications that your physician may prescribe that encourage skin healing while antibiotics can be provided to patients with infections.

If you have a wound, avoid sitting or lying on ring-shaped cushions as these tend to restrict blood flow to the surrounding tissue. Use pillows and specialty foam cushions for pressure relief on existing or potential wounds. Diet also can play an active part in wound healing, so if the patient is unable to eat or has a diet low in calories or nutrients, it will not matter how well the wound itself is treated. Good nutrition is a necessary component for wound healing and should be addressed by the physician, nurse or dietitian.

Prevention

Preventative measures need to be initiated for any patient that is at risk for pressure ulcer development. That includes frequent re-positioning to avoid tissue damage. Proper techniques need to be implemented when moving the patient as this will also reduce the risk for shearing and friction. Eat a well balanced diet to keep your skin healthy. Apply moisturizing lotions if skin is too dry, but avoid having the skin in moist areas like wet or soiled briefs for long periods of time. The skin needs be clean and dry to stay healthy. Examine pressure points frequently for those on bedrest or patients that are wheelchair bound, noting any changes in skin color.

For patients with conditions like diabetes, incontinence, circulation conditions or impaired mental status, assistance with the assessment for pressure ulcers may be necessary every day. For those patients that are immobile, range-of-motion exercise can even be beneficial.

While at the hospital, make sure to move around if possible on your own. For those patients that are unable to move on their own, a frequent turning rotation needs to be initiated by the healthcare staff. The use of pillows, foam pads and/or specialty mattresses should be in place not only for the patient with pressure ulcers, but also for those at risk for developing them.

Pressure Ulcer Considerations:
1. Prevention measures need to be implemented for all at-risk patients.
2. If sores develop, contact your physician for an evaluation.
3. All healthcare providers need to wash their hands before and after wound care.
4. Healthcare providers should also wear gloves when treating or evaluating wounds.
5. Dressings need to be changed as directed to reduce infection risk.
6. Patients need to be repositioned every two hours while on best rest.
7. Pillows, mattresses and foam pads need to be utilized for patients with pressure ulcers and those at high risk.
8. Wounds need proper assessment and individualized treatments designed for the stage of the wound and the patient's condition.
9. Eat a balanced and healthy diet.
10. Be patient, as wound healing can take a very long time.
11. Avoid ring-shaped cushions.
12. Utilize proper techniques when moving patients to reduce friction or shearing.

Sepsis

This condition develops when an infection goes systemic, or spreads to the blood stream. It can be caused by either the body's response to fighting off an infection or it can be caused by the toxic substances that the bacteria, virus or fungus are producing. According to

Sepsis.com, more than 750,000 patients are diagnosed with sepsis each year, and as many as 215,000 of those will die. It can be caused from something as minor as an untreated cut that develops an infection, or a patient with a compromised immune system, that cannot fight an infection off. Inappropriate antibiotic use has made strains of bacteria that do not respond to the general antibiotics and may have created situations that are right for this condition to develop.

Signs and Symptoms

Sepsis is a critical condition with symptoms of fever, rapid heart rate, rapid respirations, decrease blood pressure or blood flow to major organs. The patient can also exhibit symptoms of confusion or disorientation. Some may show up at the hospital with a reddish colored rash or dots throughout their body, or will report joint pain, which often mimics flu like symptoms. If any of these symptoms develop, seek immediate medical attention as this condition can deteriorate rapidly. Babies do not usually develop fevers shortly after birth, so if a baby develops a fever within the first 2 months of age, sepsis should be ruled out.

There was a patient that had been bit by a dog and developed flu-like symptoms a couple days later. She continued to work even though she knew there were times she felt a little confused or disorientated. She finally fainted and was taken to the emergency room where she was diagnosed with sepsis. It was a long recovery for this patient and she almost lost her feet, fingers, ears and nose because of the delay in treatment and the development of sepsis.

Treatment

At the hospital, the physician should be trying to figure out what is causing the sepsis condition. Blood, urine, sputum and possibly spinal fluid will be sent to the lab for evaluation because they want to identify the location of the causative agent. There may also be chest X-rays or CT scans performed to assist with the identification process. The patient will probably be on a heart monitor to continually assess their rate and rhythm. A broad spectrum antibiotic is usually prescribed until they get the specific results, and then the antibiotic may be changed. Corticosteroid treatment may be a beneficial treatment for those in septic shock. If the patient is experiencing low blood pressure, vasopressor drugs are usually administered, along with oxygen and aggressive fluid intake. The patient's blood sugar will be closely monitored and regulated within an acceptable range, and drugs to reduce a fever may also be provided. They will constantly monitor all organ function and provide the necessary treatment to prevent organ failure. Removing the causative agent such as PICC lines, urinary catheters or draining abscesses could also assist in reversing the septic shock. If necrosis occurs, amputation of extremities may be necessary to save the patient's life.

Someone with sepsis should expect to be in the ICU as this condition is critical and can carry up to an 80 percent death rate for the elderly with a compromised immune system. For a generally healthy patient, the death rate drops to around 5 percent. The recovery outcome depends on how fast the symptoms were reported and treatment was initiated. For the elderly population with some dementia already, the symptoms may go over looked, which will delay the treatment. It is always better to be seen by a physician and have them tell you it is "nothing", than to have the physician say "if you had only come in sooner, we could have done more".

Prevention

Preventative measures include tending to any cuts or scraps with a thorough cleansing, antibiotic ointment and bandages. Be sure you contact your physician if you have experienced any animal bits as they can carry bacteria in their mouth, which could lead to sepsis. If you have had surgery, make sure to wash your hands thoroughly and keep bandages intact. Consult with your physician about receiving pneumonia and flu vaccines, which could assist with health promotion. Obtain prompt medical attention if you develop any serious infections or sepsis symptoms.

Stroke

This condition is caused by either a blockage or rupture in a blood vessel in your brain. Each scenario has different risk factors and they are also treated differently. A stroke can range from very mild to very debilitating or even death. Let's talk about an ischemic stroke (a blockage) first.

A clot can develop in the blood vessel or it can originate somewhere else and travel to the brain. I once took care of a patient that was having repetitive "mini strokes" in the back of her brain. It took some time to figure out the origin, but we were able to diagnose a heart valve problem, which was caused by dental infections. There was a plaque-like build up on her heart valve, and after a while the plaque would break off, and travel to her brain causing a blockage in the blood vessels causing a stroke. The stroke that occurs due to a blockage is the most common type occurring in 8 out of 10 stroke patients.

The stroke with a "bleed" or hemorrhage develops when there is a leak or rupture in an artery in the brain. This type occurs less frequently but often has more deadly results. In the United States, Strokes are the 3rd leading cause of death with an estimated 160,000 of those patients dying each year. There are about 700,000 stroke patients each year, but the CDC has found that some states could have almost double the prevalence of strokes than others. Understand the signs and symptoms of a stroke can facilitate early treatment, which is necessary for this condition.

Signs and Symptoms

Patients often show signs of numbness or weakness on one side. The patient's speech can be slurred or garbled. The vision changes can present with the patient reporting trouble seeing, double or blurry vision. They may also be confused, have trouble walking, a severe headache or even be unconsciousness. If you or a loved one is experiencing any of these symptoms, you need to call 911 right away. This is a condition where you want to be at the top of the emergency room's list.

The last thing you want to do is come to the hospital and sit in the waiting room if you are having a stroke. With a stroke, every second counts as there are treatments that need to start within a short period of time after experiencing a stroke, and one variable in your recovery may depend on how soon the treatment is started. It is also important to know what your local hospitals specialize in, as some are Centers of Excellence for treating stroke patients.

My father-in-law, had a mild stroke several years ago, so he is still at risk for another one. He lives right in the middle of two hospitals, but one is a Stroke Center of Excellence. He could go to the hospital that can offer stroke evaluation (which is actually done by a physician via television monitors from another hospital), or he could just go directly to the hospital that has the Stroke Center of Excellence. If he needs an intervention he would need to be transferred to the stroke center anyway. In emergency situations, you may not always have a choice of hospitals depending on where you live or what the circumstances are. Be prepared and when you have an emergency you will know where to go for treatment.

A local hospital advertises that "choosing the right hospital may be the most important decision you ever make". As this may be true, I am an advocate for my patients to make sure that they are making informed decisions. You want to go where you can get the best care for your condition.

Treatment

Stroke patients should be taken to a hospital where they should expect to have an assessment, CT scan of the brain and laboratory studies to confirm the diagnosis. The CT will usually show the problem area, but there are times that it is necessary to repeat the test, as very mild strokes may not show up.

For a stroke with a clot, there can be medications utilized in your treatment, but certain parameters need to be met. If it has been less than three hours from the beginning of the symptoms, the medication tPA can be administered and have a dramatic affect on dissolving the clot. The difficulty in administering this drug is knowing when the stroke started.

With my Father-in-law's stroke, he was talking to a friend on the phone when his speech began to slur. We knew exactly when it started, but we do not always have that luxury. Patients today may also have many other conditions that practitioners need to address as well as the stroke and these conditions can play an active role in the type of treatment the patient receives.

If the patient has a bleeding problem, the physician will need to weigh the risks against the benefits before starting tPA, as it could cause other complications. This is a very serious problem and you need to put your life in the hands of experienced physicians.

There may be times that it is necessary for the physician to do a surgical procedure that removes the clot. Here again, there are risks associated with this treatment, but it may also save your life. The risks need to be weighed against the benefits.

If the stroke entails a rupture or leak in a blood vessel, it may be necessary to surgically repair it. The doctors may need to administer medications that control the brain swelling, blood pressure or other conditions. Depending on the type, severity, response to treatment and other complications, your hospital stay could range from just a trip to the emergency room, to a long stay in the hospital or rehabilitation facility. With both types of stroke, there is always the possibility of the patient never coming home.

Once the patient's condition stabilizes they may be sent for rehabilitation at a facility that specializes in stroke patients. Here the recovery effort will be focused on regaining the function that was lost due to the stroke. Depending on the patient's condition, this may take weeks, months or years. There is also the possibility that pre-stroke function levels will never be totally regained. Physicians cannot tell how much function will be regained; it is always just a wait and see response.

Prevention

Stroke prevention can often be obtained by managing your high blood pressure, high cholesterol and diabetes. Remember the alternative treatments mentioned previously for these conditions as they can be effective condition modifiers. Prevention can also include smoking cessation and avoiding secondhand smoke, as those that smoke are twice as likely to have a stroke. Maintaining a proper diet of fruits, grains, fish and decreased salt intake can lower the risk for plaque build up in the arteries.

Aspirin and garlic can also have a beneficial effect, but you need to check with your doctor prior to starting a new regiment, including holistic treatments. Garlic can have a blood thinning effect, which could be dangerous with a bleeding stroke. Always carry a list of your medications and herbal supplements with you, as your doctor may not remember what medications you are taking. Additional stroke information can be found at:

http://www.stroke.org
http://www.strokecenter.org/

Ulcers

There are millions of people with this condition and some will end up in the hospital due to complications. An ulcer is like a sore in the digestive tract, and if untreated can lead to bleeding, or a perforation in the digestive tract lining. If a perforation occurs, the contents of the digestive tract are now being leaked into the abdominal cavity. Most patients with a perforated ulcer will end up at the hospital. Depending on how long the perforation has been there will factor into the treatment and recovery time. Understanding the causative factors can help with prevention and treatment.

It used to be thought that spicy food or stress was the reason for ulcer development, but today, doctors believe that most peptic ulcers are caused by a bacterial infection or some medications. The Helicobacter pylori (H-pylori) bacteria are thought to be the major culprit of ulcers, and can be confirmed by a biopsy of the affected area.

Excessive acid production, smoking, stress, alcohol and taking nonsteroidal anti-inflammatory drugs (NSAIDs) which can cause an irritation of the stomach or intestine lining and can all increase the risk for ulcer development. It is estimated that around 10 percent of the American population will develop an ulcer over their lifetime so let's look at the different types of ulcers.

The different ulcer types are provided names for the various locations in which the ulcers are commonly found. If an ulcer occurs in the stomach, it is called a gastric ulcer, while those in the small intestines are called a duodenal ulcer. Ulcers in your esophagus are called esophageal ulcers and usually are caused by acid reflux disease.

Signs and Symptoms

The signs and symptoms of an ulcer can vary with location and the extent of the disease, but many patients experience sharp, burning pain in the abdomen, ranging from their breastbone to their navel. With duodenal (intestinal) ulcers, the pain usually occurs within a few hours after eating. If the pain is relieved by eating or taking an antacid, a duodenal ulcer could be present.

If the pain is caused by eating and not relieved with antacid treatment, you may have a gastric ulcer. Pain is the general symptom of ulcers, but the patient can experience nausea, vomiting, changes in stool color and unexplained weight loss. The symptoms may wax and wane as the stomach acid comes in contact with the ulcer.

Treatment

In order to diagnosis this condition, most physicians will want to look at your esophagus, stomach and the upper portion of your small intestines to confirm their suspicions. This is usually performed under a mild sedation in the physician's office or the hospital. If an ulcer is found, it is generally biopsied for tissue examination.

Treatment for mild ulcers is usually managed with medications like acid blockers. They reduce the hydrochloric acid your body produces which can reduce the pain, and encourage the ulcer to heal. Some of these medications can be bought over the counter or as a prescription. Antibiotics may be necessary if H. pylori is discovered, and may be used in combination with other medications.

For peptic ulcers, physicians can also prescribe proton pump inhibitors which also reduce acid as their main course of action. If you have a bleeding ulcer, it may be necessary for intravenous treatment, to allow for "healing time" of the ulcerative area. Some medications for ulcer treatment are designed to "coat" the stomach and small intestines which also can encourage healing. If the ulcer fails to heal, more rigorous treatment measures may be necessary, but surgery is utilized only as a last resort. The surgeon's experience, the location of the perforation and the patient's condition will all be considered when developing a treatment plan. The patient's hospital stay could consist of maybe a day or two for minor ulcers to maybe a week if bowel surgery is necessary. It all depends on the individual patient's condition.

Prevention

The underlining cause needs to be addressed if you have been diagnosed with any type of ulcer, which may include a modification in your daily activities like smoking cessation or stress reduction. Smokers have double the risk for developing ulcers, and alcohol consumption has also been linked to worsen ulcers or increase pain, so monitor your participation in these behaviors.

Work with the physician to find your ulcer's cause, but this may take some detective work and time, so be patient. The condition did not occur over night, and may take a little while for it to subside.

CHAPTER 4

Hospital Infectious Diseases

We have all read the headlines or heard the news reports of disease outbreaks of one kind or another, but have you ever really thought about it when you go to the hospital? Most people would like to think about the hospital making them well or providing services in a sterile environment.

We often picture the hospital with bright white lab coats, sterile gloves and a recently sanitized stethoscope, right? How about those crisp white sheets, the sparkling clean restroom, or your cheerful roommate in the bed beside you, that keeps coughing all night long? Do you know if the housekeeper cleaned your bed and table enough to kill all the germs that were on it from the previous patient? How about the water supply, your nurses' scrubs or your doctor's cell phone?

All of these things can carry disease that can put your life at risk. A recent study published in *Infection Control and Hospital Epidemiology*, reported that healthcare workers had "picked up" a significant pathogen, like VRE or MRSA, 53 percent of the time after touching a surface around the patient. If the healthcare worker did not wash their hands, the pathogen can be "carried" to the next patient. Only in the perfect world would we find uncompromised, germ-proof conditions at a hospital. What the healthcare workers are "carrying" or your hospital bed is "covered in", could make you deathly sick and even cost you your life.

Hospitals are in the business of returning you to health, but every year there are 1.75 to 3.5 million patients that are admitted to hospitals in the United States and somewhere around 10 percent of those will contract nosocomial (hospital acquired) infections.

The Centers for Disease Control (CDC) reports that around 90,000 of those patients with nosocomial infections will die this year alone. These statistics ranks nosocomial infections as one of the leading causes of death in a hospital setting. This is an astounding number considering diseases like; Heart Disease, Cancer, Stroke and Pneumonia are also on that list.

As a visitor, the objects you touch or the air you breathe can also put your life at risk, as well as your family's. If you carry the "bugs" home you could be infecting anyone else that you come in contact with. There has been recent concern over hospital employees wearing their scrubs to other places after they have worked at the hospital. The potential for contamination truly exists. There are situations that you need to consider prior to your hospital visit, no matter if you are a patient or a visitor.

Staying Healthy

First and foremost try to stay healthy. Prevention is one key element that you have control over. Exercise, proper diet and rest can all have a great impact on your health. For example, studies have shown a direct correlation with a low fat diet reducing the risk for coronary artery disease, which can lead to heart attacks or strokes. Knowing your family history can assist you with making modifications that can alter your familiar health history. My mother had cancer when I was 20 years old and I was told then that I am at high risk for developing this as well. They told my mother 25 years ago to buy organic meats and watch her caffeine intake, so I changed my habits 20 years sooner than my mother did. I practice

HOSPITAL INFECTIOUS DISEASES

other preventative measures, but you must know what you are at risk for, and how you can modify those risk factors. Although researchers think that there may be genetic reasons for diseases repeating from one generation to another, there are other factors such the same diet, environmental exposures and life style habits that contribute to this pattern as well.

We are faced daily with diseases, and our body is able to ward them off, most of the time. One easy thing anyone can do to help reduce the risk for infection is hand washing. We touch so many things after someone else has just wiped their nose, coughed into their hand or tended to other bodily fluids. We cannot rely on someone else to protect us, so wash your hands to prevent the spread of disease.

I will never forget a hospital meeting where there were bagels provided on a tray in the middle of the table. One person came in and picked almost all of them up before she decided to take the one on the bottom. Now the rest of the people sitting at the table were all nurses and I know thought the same thing..."I can't believe she just touched all of those". Needless to say, no one else really wanted to eat the bagels after she had handled them all. We worked in a hospital where germs grow everywhere and you do not know what is growing on the door handles, elevator buttons or the cafeteria tables. Hand washing is the first line of defense, but also consider who's hands or mouth has been on the food you are about to eat.

Clemson University did a recent study on double dipping and the contamination that occurs when this happens. Good bacteria are not harmful, but if someone is toting bad bacteria, beware. A good rule of thumb is unless you are willing to use that person's toothbrush, you might think twice about eating the dip after someone has double-dipped their favorite veggie.

It always concerns me when I go in a fast food restaurant and see a sign in the bathroom that says "all employees are required to wash their hands". I am not sure if that is put there to make me feel better or if I should just take it as a reminder to the staff. My mind often wanders and considers if they have to be reminded about that, what else they are forgetting.

Safe food handling has been in the news lately with outbreaks of E-Coli and Salmonella being reported across the nation. Some of these outbreaks have cost millions of dollars in lost of product but there is no comparison to the cost of the lives that have been lost because of these outbreaks. We must consider that all food could possibly harbor bacteria or other contaminants. Wash everything thoroughly and make sure to prevent cross contamination of raw meats and other foods. Consider your utensils as they come in contact with raw meat and either wash the utensil, or use a clean one to serve the meat once it is done cooking. It only takes one case of food poisoning for you to take preventative measures the next time, and those that have lost their life over it, will not be able to have that chance.

Preventative Actions

Another preventative action would be to limit your exposure to the diseases that are out there. Many diseases we do not even know we are exposed to until it is too late, but others we do. I have seen people come to the hospital with their two week old baby to see Grandma who is in the ICU with pneumonia. I know it is important to see Grandma, but you could be putting your baby's life at risk if he develops pneumonia.

Patients need family support and I strongly recommend that you have someone there most of the time if for no other reason than to have another set of eyes and ears that understand what is going on with your care, but the exposure may come at a cost. If your health is compromised in any way, do not come to the hospital where you could be exposed to even more disease. Children and the elderly are also at higher risk for developing infections and should only visit the hospital when absolutely necessary. If you do visit, make sure to limit your exposure, wash your hands, and make sure you know what condition the patient has been diagnosed with.

Conditions change from one day to the next, so check with the nursing staff or family prior to making that hospital visit, to make sure the patient's condition has not changed. It is very common to receive lab results several days after the patient has been admitted, as cultures sometimes take a while to obtain, and then the lab must let them "grow", so the process slows down the confirmed diagnosis. Just be aware that the patient could have something contagious without having a confirmed diagnosis.

I once took care of a patient that was being tested for TB. I walked into the isolation room and found the patient's daughter in the room without a mask. The difficult situation was that the daughter had been told to wear a mask, but she ignored the instruction. Although she might not have been concerned about her own health, situations like this can also put those around you in jeopardy if you develop the disease.

The patient ended up not having TB, but had the results been different, the daughter had just exposed herself and potentially others to a possible life threatening condition. I recommend that you just consider everyone in the hospital as having "something" contagious and act accordingly. Realize that the physician that just changed your bandages just walked out of your room, and may not have washed his hands, then touched the elevator button or door knob. This happens, so be proactive and protect yourself by washing your hands. You do not need to panic or become a germ-a-phobia, but a wise consumer will consider the possibility of organisms living anywhere and will take the appropriate actions.

Evaluating the hospital's infection rate online may not be 100 percent accurate, but it is a place to start. Many hospitals learn from their mistakes while others take a proactive stance against nosocomial infections. To effectively prevent nosocomial infections, the hospital should have a systematic, multidisciplinary approach in place. Surveillance of diseases, outbreak management, and implementation of protocols for the staff, patients and visitors will all be factors in an effective prevention plan.

Studies have shown that when surgeons are provided their infection rates compared to other surgeons' rates, the whole institution infection rate drops. Continual education of the hospital staff for prevention of nosocomial infections can also reduce infection rates. It is necessary for the staff to have all the essential equipment such as gown, gloves, mask, sterile equipment and cleaners if an infection-control program is going to be effective. Surveillance of the staff also puts pressure on them to maintain high standards of care. If you know that there is a policeman waiting with his radar gun a mile up the road, you are more apt to "go the speed limit". If the staff is observed and corrective action taken for non-compliant individuals, the infection rate can drop. Research shows that health care providers only wash their hands effectively about 50 percent of the time, so you have a 50-50 chance that your healthcare provider will bring you something more than your medication!

Regulations for Hospitals

There have been recent movements across the United States to require a reporting system of hospital acquired infections. The CDC estimates that around 20 billion dollars are spent each year on nosocomial type infections. A patient that came in for a knee replacement, that would have required a stay over night, now turned into a 20 day hospital stay once she contracted C.diff. She required an ICU bed for numerous days which was costly for Medicare, the hospital and the patient, not including what it did to her health.

Finally individual States, Consumer Advocates, Insurers, along with the Federal Government are starting to take notice of these situations and are taking matters into their own hands. Many States have adopted laws that require the hospitals to publicly report hospital acquired infections while others are looking into certain mandates. Prevention methods are also being adopted as the public begins to question regulations related to nosocomial infections.

Some infections can be difficult to prevent, but those hospitals that have implemented best practice policies such as strict hand hygiene, proper sanitization of rooms and equipment, assessment of possible bacteria and screening of patients prior to admission; have lowered their infection rates to nearly nothing. Some insurance companies are also refusing to pay for these hospital- acquired infections, so the hospitals will be left with "the bill" for the infections that could have been prevented. With hospitals feeling the public scrutiny, they also want to put their best foot forward, so expect to see changes implemented across the country.

Although regulations are changing daily, here is some of the most recent data organized by The Kaiser Family Foundation at http://www.statehealthfacts.org/comparetable.jsp?cat=8&ind=407&typ=5&gsa=1 for each state, and how the nosocomial infections are reported.

State	Hospital-Based Infections Reporting Requirement	Notes
	26 Yes	
Alabama	No	N/A
Alaska	No	N/A
Arizona	No	N/A
Arkansas	Yes	Health facilities must collect data on healthcare-associated infection rates; facilities may voluntarily submit quarterly reports to the Department of Health on the health facility's healthcare-associated infection rates.
California	Yes	The Healthcare Associated Infection Advisory Committee shall make recommendations for phasing in the implementation and public reporting of additional process measures and outcome measures by January 1, 2008, and, in doing so, shall consider the measures recommended by the CDC.
Colorado	Yes	Beginning July 31, 2007, health facilities required to routinely submit its hospital-acquired infection data to the national healthcare safety network in accordance with national healthcare safety network requirements and procedures.
Connecticut	Yes	By October 2007 Department of Public Health required to have mandatory reporting system for healthcare associated infections and appropriate standardized measures for the reporting of data related to healthcare associated infections.

Delaware	Yes	Hospitals must submit quarterly reports on their hospital-acquired infection rates to the Department of Health and Social Services using the accepted Centers for Disease Control and Prevention's (CDC) National Healthcare Safety Network ("NHSN") definitions.
District of Columbia	No	N/A
Florida	Yes	Health care facilities must electronically report data on hospital-acquired infections to Agency for Healthcare Administration, as specified in regulations.
Georgia	No	N/A
Hawaii	No	N/A
Idaho	No	N/A
Illinois	Yes	Infection rates to be reported to state Department of Healthcare and Family Services.
Indiana	Yes	A health care facility, a health care professional, or an individual may file with state patient safety data agency reports relating to hospital-acquired infections.
Iowa	No	N/A
Kansas	No	N/A
Kentucky	No	N/A
Louisiana	No	N/A
Maine	No	N/A
Maryland	Yes	Health care-associated infection information from hospitals to be reported to state
Massachusetts	No	N/A
Michigan	No	N/A
Minnesota	No	By January 1, 2009, the Minnesota Hospital Association shall develop a Web-based system for reporting hospital-specific performance on public reporting measures for hospital-acquired infections.
Mississippi	Yes	N/A
Missouri	Yes	The state shall collect data annually on required nosocomial infection incidence rates from hospitals, ambulatory surgical centers, and other facilities; Medical facilities must also report nosocomial infection outbreaks (FN 1)
Montana	No	N/A

HOSPITAL INFECTIOUS DISEASES

Nebraska	Yes	Each hospital licensed in Nebraska shall, at least annually, provide surgeons performing surgery at such hospital a report as to the number and rates of surgical infections in surgical patients of such surgeon; Health care providers must also report to a patient safety organization all unanticipated deaths or major permanent losses of function associated with health care associated nosocomial infection
Nevada	Yes	Within 14 days of the occurrence, a health care facility must report the date, the time and a brief description of the event to the state health division
New Hampshire	Yes	Each hospital shall regularly report to the department the hospital infection data it has collected, including data on central line related bloodstream infections, ventilator associated pneumonia, surgical wound infections, and urinary tract infections
New Jersey	Yes	A health care entity shall maintain for a period of four years all records and source data relating to its infection rate and shall make the records available to the division, the board which licenses or otherwise authorizes the health care professional, the review panel and the Department of Health and Senior Services, as applicable, upon request
New Mexico	No	N/A
New York	Yes	Each general hospital shall maintain a program capable of identifying and tracking hospital acquired infections for the purpose of public reporting under this section and quality improvement. Each hospital shall regularly report to the department the hospital infection data it has collected. (FN 2)
North Carolina	No	N/A
North Dakota	No	N/A
Ohio	Yes	Hospitals must report volume of infections to director of health.
Oklahoma	Yes	For device-related blood stream infections, hospitals must report to the Hospital Advisory Council.
Oregon	No	N/A
Pennsylvania	Yes	Providers must submit to the Health Care Cost Containment Council rates of infection for specified diagnoses and treatments, grouped by severity, for individual providers.
Rhode Island	Yes	Infection outbreaks (as defined by the department of health via regulation) shall be reported to the department of health division of facilities regulation.

South Carolina	Yes	Hospitals shall submit reports at least every six months on their hospital acquired infection rates to the Department of Health. Reports must be submitted in a format and at a time as provided for by the department. These reports must be made available to the public at each hospital and through the department. The first report must be submitted before February 1, 2008.
South Dakota	No	N/A
Tennessee	Yes	Every facility shall report unusual events, and certain other defined incidents, to the department of health within seven (7) business days from the facility's identification of the event or incident. These events include intravascular catheter related events including necrosis or infection requiring repair. Most facilities must also report infections to the Centers for Disease Control's National Nosocomial Infection Surveillance/National Healthcare Safety Network (NNIS/NHSN) surveillance system.
Texas	Yes	Health care facilities must report certain enumerated health care-associated infections to the Texas Department of Health. The department shall ensure that the health care-associated infections a health care facility is required to report have the meanings assigned by the federal Centers for Disease Control and Prevention.
Utah	No	N/A
Vermont	Yes	Health Care Commissioner shall adopt rules establishing a standard format for community reports, as well as the contents, which shall include measures of hospital-acquired infections that are valid, reliable, and useful, including comparisons to appropriate industry benchmarks.
Virginia	Yes	Acute care hospitals shall report information about nosocomial infections to the Centers for Disease Control and Prevention's National Healthcare Safety Network. Such hospitals shall release their infection data to the Board of Health. The specific infections to be reported, the hospitals required to report, and patient populations to be included shall be prescribed by Board regulation. (effective July 1, 2008)

HOSPITAL INFECTIOUS DISEASES

Washington	Yes	Hospitals must collect and report data related to the following health care-associated infections: beginning July 1, 2008, central line-associated bloodstream infection in the intensive care unit; beginning January 1, 2009, ventilator-associated pneumonia; and beginning January 1, 2010, surgical site infection for the following procedures: deep sternal wound for cardiac surgery, including coronary artery bypass graft; total hip and knee replacement surgery; and hysterectomy, abdominal and vaginal. Hospitals must routinely collect and submit the data to the national healthcare safety network of the United States centers for disease control and prevention in accordance with national healthcare safety network definitions, methods, requirements, and procedures.
West Virginia	No	N/A
Wisconsin	No	N/A
Wyoming	No	N/A

The Kaiser Family Foundation, statehealthfacts.org. March 1, 2009 *Reprint with permission of Kaiser Foundation*

It is recommend that you review how your state is regulated, and if it is not up to par, contact your State Representatives and let them know how you feel. Hospital acquired infections can have devastating affects on one's health, and thousands will even lose their life because they have contacted this type of condition. Even though patients come to the hospital for elective surgery, they are still at risk for developing a nosocomial (hospital acquired) infection. No one is exempt.

Today we are faced with some of the toughest "super bugs" that render our normal antibiotic regiments helpless. Weakened immune systems, chronic diseases, along with the overuse of antibiotics, have all made us more susceptible to these bacteria. Understanding what these diseases are and how to avoid them can provide protection from potentially fatal conditions.

The hospital is a place where "sick" people go and take all of their diseases with them. Over the next few pages we will discuss what diseases you could be exposed to and what things you can do to prevent it from occuring.

For more information about hospital acquired infections you can research the websites listed below:

www.stophospitalinfections.org. Information on state laws.
www.hospitalinfection.org Provided by the Committee to Reduce Infection Deaths.
www.shea-online.org is the Society for Healthcare Epidemiology of America.
www.leapfroggroup.org provides infection rating for 1300 U.S. hospitals.

General considerations for disease prevention:
1. Wash your hands, wash your hands, and wash your hands.
2. Do not come to the hospital if you are sick or have a compromised immune system.
3. Do not bring babies and young children to visit patients at the hospital unless necessary.
4. Know what the patient's condition is before visiting.
5. If the patient has an isolation sign on the door, check with the nurse for instructions.
6. Assume that everyone in the hospital is contagious.
7. After you leave the hospital wash your hands and your clothes to protect yourself and those around you.
8. Reference websites for your state's regulations.
9. Find out what your local hospital's infection rate is at www.healthgrades.com.
10. Protect cuts and wounds with antibiotic ointment and a bandage.
11. Realize that alcohol based hand sanitizers do not kill all bacteria in the hospital setting.

Methicillin-resistant Staphylococcus Aureus (MRSA)

Staph aureus has been a common hospital acquired infection for a long time, but there is a new strain that has come to the forefront over the last few decades called MRSA. This acronym stands for methicillin-resistant staphylococcus aureus, which is a bacteria that is resistant to most broad-spectrum antibiotics (the drugs we used to treat most infections). This medication resistant strain was first reported around 1947, but was not reported in the United States until 1968. MRSA is responsible for about 52 percent of all staph aureus nosocomial infections. Most cases will develop in the hospital or shortly after a hospital visit, but the condition is being reported more commonly in the community as well. Community acquired MRSA (CA-MRSA) generally is reported in skin conditions. The CA-MRSA has been found in places where whirlpools, showers, tables and exercise equipment are shared in a community-like setting. More cases of CA-MRSA are reported all the time and schools along with major sports teams have found it necessary to totally disinfect their locker rooms because outbreaks of CA-MRSA have occurred.

Anyone can develop MRSA but those with a compromised immune system, which is common in most patients in the hospital, are more susceptible. MRSA can develop anywhere in the body, but is generally found in the blood stream, surgical wounds, respiratory tract, heart, bones and skin. The staph bacterial can be found on your skin and in your nose without any noticeable symptoms in healthy people, but still could be spread to others.

Overuse of antibiotics has made the bacteria become resistant to commonly used medications, so it is recommended to only take antibiotics when necessary. Many people pressure their doctors to prescribe an antibiotic every time they are sick, but the antibiotics do not work for viruses. Antibiotics can cure an infection, but even when used appropriately, they can still set us up for developing a resistant strain of bacteria. To prevent unnecessary antibiotic treatments, your doctor needs to know if you have a virus or a bacterial infection prior to treatment initiation. Humans are not the only ones that take antibiotics that could create drug resistant organisms.

Livestock are also injected with antibiotics, and then are brought into our food chain, and into our bodies. The end result has also been bacteria that are resistant to many medications. Transmission of the infection comes in several different methods. Look for those packages of meat that say "antibiotic free" to be proactive in reducing drug resistant bacteria in our food chain.

How MRSA is transmitted depends on where it is located. If it is in the blood, wounds, skin or urine, it is transmitted by contact. If you have a cut or scrape and come in contact with this type of MRSA you could be at risk of developing the infection. It is always important to cover any cuts or wounds with medicated ointment and a bandage as MRSA can live on surfaces for hours or even months.

When visiting a patient with the "contact" form of MRSA, you should wear a gown (they are provided by the hospital) over your clothes to prevent your clothes from coming in contact with the infection, and gloves if you are going to touch the infected patient's items. There is always a concern over contaminated items at the hospital, and we need to be aware of what those items could be for effective prevention.

One hospital that I worked in randomly had someone performing surveillance of the staff to see if they washed their hands appropriately. One surveyor was upset the nursing assistant had not washed her hands in between taking each patient's blood pressure. I agreed that she should have done that, but I also reminded the surveyor that the nursing assistant used the same blood pressure cuff from one person to another. In this case the blood pressure cuff came in more contact with the patient than the nursing assistant. There is the chance of MRSA "living" on items in the hospital which include the healthcare provider's hands, linens, night stands, bed rails, restrooms, blood pressure cuffs, clothes and stethoscopes. Even your doctor's coat and tie could be carrying the disease. Because we cannot see the bacteria, the possibilities of where MRSA could be living are endless.

We take care of patients at the hospital all the time with MRSA and it is has almost reached the point that many healthcare providers do not blink twice with a MRSA diagnosis. Healthcare workers do not intentionally try to infect patients, but they need to make sure they are taking every precaution necessary to prevent it. There is nothing wrong with asking a healthcare provider to wash their hands and wear gloves prior to touching you.

There have been cases where a patient has been discharged from the hospital and the lab work comes back positive for an infectious disease, but the healthcare providers, visitors or roommates had no idea that the patient had this condition. Remember, paranoia is not the objective, but you need to conduct your actions appropriately for the situation you are in. A "contact" type infection is a little easier to contain, but respiratory MRSA can be in the air.

If MRSA is in the respiratory tract, it could be transmitted through the sputum or the air. Wearing a mask and gown while visiting an infected patient can protect you from being exposed to the bacteria. If the MRSA is not respiratory related, a gown and gloves should be sufficient protection.

Patients in the hospital have an increased risk for MRSA just because their exposure time is greater, and according to the CDC the risk dramatically increases if the patient's stay is over 14 days. The average patient will see at least one doctor, two to three nurses and two to three nursing assistants every day. Your room mate, dieticians, transporters, lab technicians, etc., could all provide you some form of service while in the hospital, but they see most of the other patients in the hospital as well. Patients are often given the option to stay an "extra day" for one reason or another, but for every day that you stay in the hospital, your risk for contracting a super-bug goes higher.

The ICU has been of much focus when it comes to infectious diseases. Patients in the ICU generally have multiple conditions which put them at greater risk of developing an infection like MRSA. Ventilator-associated pneumonia (VAP) is one of the most horrendous infections that can affect a hospitalized patient, and even more so if the bacteria is MRSA. There is a clear association with VAP and morbidity but new preventative measures have shown promise in reducing these infections.

Proper hand washing has also reduced infection rates in the ICU at facilities that have adopted these infection prevention protocols. Here again it is appropriate for you to ask about what prevention protocols your local hospital participates in. Remember that they want your business, so make sure they are doing everything possible, for when you do need their services.

Symptoms

Signs and symptoms of MRSA depends on the location and can range from a small skin infection like cellulitis, boils, abscesses or a sty, to more severe symptoms like fever, joint pain, headaches, low blood pressure, rash, coughing or shortness of breath, which all need immediate medical attention. If you have been in a hospital, nursing home facility, around patients with MRSA or in a community setting such as gyms or locker rooms and develop these symptoms, contact your primary physician, or go to your local emergency room for evaluation.

Treatment

MRSA is usually treated with the antibiotics Vancomycin or Zyvox, but there are cases of MRSA that are becoming resistant even to Vancomycin. Mupirocin antibiotic creams can also be used to help eliminate MRSA colonization from the mucous membranes. An antibiotic regiment may take from 14-28 days. If you are receiving an IV antibiotic, you will probably have a PICC line which stands for: peripherally inserted central venous catheter. This type of catheter is inserted into your smaller blood vessels, but is long enough to reach to your larger blood vessels. With a PICC line, the medication can enter the body through larger blood vessels which can reduce the irritation these strong medications can have on the smaller veins. The medications play an important part in eradicating these bacteria, so it is important to finish all of the medication as prescribed. It is possible to recover from MRSA, but the laboratory results will be needed to confirm this.

MRSA prevention considerations:
1. Wash your hands regularly with antimicrobial soap.
2. Limit your exposure to the hospital and those diagnosed with MRSA.
3. Remember that bacteria could be living anywhere at the hospital.

HOSPITAL INFECTIOUS DISEASES

4. Take preventative measures such as gowns, gloves and masks when working with MRSA patients or high risk situations.
5. Make sure all healthcare providers wash their hands prior to touching you.
6. Clean surfaces and equipment with a disinfectant that is effective against MRSA. A tablespoon of bleach in 1 quart of water will provide the necessary disinfectant for killing MRSA. You will find a list of products effective against MRSA at http://epa.gov/oppad001/list_h_mrsa_vre.pdf.
7. Limit items taken to the hospital to prevent contamination.
8. Clothes and linens that may carry MRSA will need to be washed in hot water >160 degrees Fahrenheit. Commercial dryers also provide enough heat that will kill the bacteria.
9. Avoid community locker rooms and equipment. Exercise at home.
10. Protect cuts and wounds with antibiotic ointment and a bandage.
11. If symptoms of MRSA develop, contact your physician or local emergency room.
12. Cultures should be done weekly to assess treatment effectiveness.
13. Complete the medication regiment as prescribed.

Clostridium difficile (C-Diff)

Every year about a half million Americans will be diagnosed with C-Diff, and the numbers appear to be rising around 10 percent each year, with the death rate climbing even higher. This condition seems to be increasing in virulence and is becoming more difficult to treat. C.diff can develop into a severe infection in the intestines, called pseudomembranous colitis. This condition can be life threatening, so it is also imperative to understand the whole dynamics of C.diff, for your own protection.

There are different strains of C.diff reported worldwide, and they have gone from very low numbers of reported cases, to astronomical numbers, nearly doubling between 2000 and 2005. There appears to be one "front runner" in the C.diff strains, called NAP1 here in the U.S. This particular strain showed more prevalence after it developed a resistance to fluoroquinolone antibiotics, and there is some indication that it could also be developing resistance to Flagyl, a drug often used for treatment. Approximately 300,000 patients diagnosed with C-diff will require hospitalization, and this condition actually sends more patients to the hospital each year than MRSA.

C-diff bacteria are normally found in the intestinal tract and can act as "good" bacteria, but when there is an overgrowth situation, it becomes a "bad" bacteria. Too much of a good thing is not always beneficial to your health, and when this bacteria takes over, it produces toxins that disrupt the normal flora in the colon. The toxins that are released can injure the lining of the intestines and can cause devastating results. The NAP1 strain produces 16-23 times more toxins than its cohorts, which could explain how C.diff has become difficult to treat.

Once an individual has been infected with the C.diff spores, it is unclear how soon symptoms will develop, but studies have suggested that it could take less than seven days. There are a few things that put you at risk for developing C.diff including ingestion the C.diff spores or if something has disrupted the normal bacteria in your colon. Antibiotic used to treat other infections can also kills the "good" bacteria, resulting in a C.diff over growth. Anti-ulcer medications have been associated with C.diff because they reduce the acidity of the stomach. This alteration in acid can also allow C.diff to grow uncontrolled.

If you have had a long hospital stay, your risk for developing C.diff escalates, as this condition can be readily spread from one patient to another by the health care providers or other patients. Often the patient will develop this condition while sharing a room with another patient without even knowing it. If your immune system is compromised or you are over 65 years of age, the risk for contacting C.diff also increases.

There has been some evidence that C.diff could also affect the food that we eat, but research has not proven this theory. Understanding the symptoms and treatment for this condition will assist with developing a prevention plan.

Symptoms

This condition is even more frightening than other "super bugs" due to its easy transmission and longevity. The spores produced by C.diff easily spread to surfaces including items such as toilet seats, door knobs, sink faucets, bed rails, divider curtains and can live up to five months on infected surfaces. The spores are easily transmitted when you touch one of these infected surfaces, and then transfer your hand or food to your mouth. The bacteria affects your intestinal tract and can cause symptoms of watery mucus like diarrhea, blood in the stool, fever, abdominal pain, cramping or tenderness. If the cause is related to antibiotic use, the symptoms can even show up as late as two to six weeks after you have finished the antibiotic treatment. With the rapid loss of fluids, you can also experience dehydration related to the C-diff. Many nurses report that C.diff has a certain smell about it, and has assisted with early detection of the condition. Once a nurse associates the distinct smell with C.diff, it is unforgettable, so chalk one up for the experienced nurse. If the causative agent can be removed soon after symptoms develop, it increases the patient's rate of recovery, and their chance of survival.

Treatment

If C.diff is suspected, a culture of the stool should be obtained, for an accurate diagnosis. Patients in the hospital with a confirmed diagnosis of C.diff should be in an isolation room, but could share a room with another C.diff patient if necessary.

The first line of defense is usually to discontinue any current antibiotics, and start a regiment of Flagyl or Vancomycin for 7-10 days. Oral Flagyl has a great success rate, but so often patients have other medical conditions that can cause additional complications, which can make it more difficult to gain control of the patient's recovery. With the NAP1 strain developing resistance to Flagyl, the physicians may be forced to try other medications. Probiotics can also be administered to assist with gaining a balance in the intestinal flora, and in some cases it is necessary to surgically remove part of the colon. This could result in the patient having a colostomy, depending on the location of the intestine that is removed. Make sure that you fully understand the risks not only with the condition, but with any surgical procedures prior to treatment.

Because of the great amount of fluid lost with C.diff, you will most likely be receiving IV fluids and encouraged to drink plenty of liquids unless contraindicated. Once you are able to eat, foods like saltine crackers, bananas, soup, potatoes, noodles, and other starchy foods should be encouraged, but diary products may be difficult to digest. Once diagnosed with C.diff, there is a higher chance of developing it again so let's look at ways to prevent it.

Prevention

First and foremost everyone needs to wash their hands. Spores can survive routine soaps, so thoroughly washing is required to remove them off of your hands. Alcohol based hand sanitizers will not remove C.diff, and healthcare workers or visitors should also use gloves and gowns when taking care of or visiting C.diff patients. Because the spores are resistant to most cleaners (including alcohol based), contaminated areas should be disinfected with a product that contains bleach. Curtains that divide the patient rooms should be removed after C.diff patients leave, but here again you are putting your life in someone else's hands. It might just be in your best interest to not touch the curtains in the rooms unless you are wearing gloves. Do not share towels, washcloths, toothbrushes or other hygiene items that could be infected by the C.diff patient. There is some disagreement on the exact temperature to launder infected patient's clothing and bedding in, but including bleach in the water can kill the spores.

Antibiotics should be administered only when necessary and consider eating yogurt when you do have to take them to maintain

HOSPITAL INFECTIOUS DISEASES

the flora balance of the intestines. Many antibiotics can cause diarrhea, but that does not mean that it is C-Diff. If yogurt does not help with your diarrhea, it may be necessary for you to contact your physician as, he may want to change the antibiotic regiment or discontinue it if possible. Symptoms of severe diarrhea should always be evaluated by a physician.

C.diff prevention considerations:
1. Wash hands before and after taking care of or visiting patients with C.diff.
2. C.diff lives a long time on surfaces, so assume that it could be anywhere in the hospital environment.
3. Disinfect surfaces exposed to C.diff with bleach products.
4. Do not take antibiotics unless necessary.
5. Eat yogurt to keep the flora in balance when taking antibiotics if possible.
6. Take things to the hospital that you can either throw away when you leave, or clean with bleach.
7. Wear gowns when visiting C.diff patients.
8. Wear a protective gown and gloves if providing direct care of C.diff patients.
9. Do not set your purse or belongings on the hospital floor or other areas that could be contaminated.
10. Eating utensils should not come in contact with nightstands or bedside tables.
11. Toothbrushes should not come in contact with any room furniture or sink areas, to avoid possible contamination.
12. Launder clothes appropriately when treating C.diff patients.

Hepatitis A

There are several different types of Hepatitis so let us start with Hepatitis A. This is generally a condition found in unsanitary conditions. It is usually transmitted by you putting something in your mouth that is contaminated with stool from an infected person. If the infected person does not wash their hands after using the restroom, they can carry the disease on their hands and spread it to other surfaces. We often see this in the food industry as an infected worker handles your food or drinks and then passes the disease along to you.

Symptoms and Treatment

Hepatitis A patients will generally have a poor appetite, fever, vomiting and a general weak feeling. Because all of the Hepatitis diseases affect the liver, the patient can experience dark color urine, jaundice of the skin and the whites of their eyes may turn yellow. The good news is that this condition is rarely fatal, but there is not really any treatment for the condition. Symptoms will be treated with plenty of fluids and rest, but it could take months for it to totally disappear.

Prevention

Prevention methods include a short term vaccine if visiting countries with poor sanitation. Hand washing is an easy method to prevent not only yourself from contracting the disease but also spreading it to others if you have the condition. The vaccine may also be recommended if you use illegal drugs, live in communities with high Hepatitis A rates, have homosexual relations, or live in institutions for the developmentally challenged. If you know that you have been exposed, the vaccine could prevent the disease from developing.

Hepatitis B

Hepatitis B (HBV) is an infection that affects the liver and is found in blood and bodily fluids. On average, 200,000 people come down with HBV every year and of those, close to 5,000 will die. The condition can range from a mild illness which may last a few weeks, to a long term illness, from which you many never recover. Those at greatest risk are IV drug users, those with tattoos or piercings, sharing of personal items like razors or toothbrushes and babies with mothers diagnosed with the disease. If you visit a patient in the hospital with Hepatitis, your risk for contracting the disease is low as long as you wash your hands and cover all cuts or scrapes.

Symptoms

Symptoms include feeling tired, low fever, headache, feeling sick to your stomach, diarrhea, constipation, muscle pain, joint pain or yellowing of the eyes and skin. The condition is diagnosed with blood tests as well as an assessment of your liver function.

Treatment

Treatment generally consists of eating healthy foods, avoiding alcohol and drugs, and getting proper rest. There are medications for chronic Hepatitis B, but not everyone can take these. In severe cases the condition could even render a liver transplant.

Prevention

Preventative measures include not sharing needles, razors, or toothbrushes. Wear a condom when you have sex and wear gloves if you have to touch blood or body fluids of an infected patient. There is also a vaccine that is administered in three individual doses, but reports have found that immunity is not always developed even if you have the recommended doses. A general concern over your risk for exposure can be resolved if your titers are evaluated and your immunity levels are within a protective range.

Hepatitis C

Although hepatitis in general may not seem as virulent as other diseases we have discussed, the long term affects can be devastating. Hepatitis C (HCV) is a virus that causes a liver infection and can result in damage to the liver. HCV is spread by coming in contact with someone's blood that is positive for the disease. The CDC reports that around 800 cases were reported in 2006, but admits that thousands more acquired the disease that year after reviewing underreporting analysis and those without symptoms.

Newly diagnosed patients with HCV do not usually have symptoms, so an accurate number of confirmed cases would always appear low with the methods we currently have for reporting this disease. Those individuals at greatest risk are drug users, blood transfusion recipients, organ transplant recipients prior to July 1992, hemodialysis patients, HIV patients, children born to mothers that have HCV, and healthcare workers.

Symptoms

The symptoms include fever, fatigue, dark urine, abdominal pain, nausea, vomiting, clay-colored stool, jaundice of the skin, yellowing of the eyes, and loss of appetite. It may take 4-24 weeks for the symptoms to develop, but most individuals with HCV do not develop symptoms, but may have liver disease develop including cirrhosis or liver cancer. Patients may go for years without any idea that they are infected with the disease. It is often caught when a screening is done for blood donation or an annual physical where liver enzyme levels are abnormal. HCV can go away on its own, but it is reported in a low percentage of patients and the medical community does not know what makes it go away at this time.

Treatment

Treatment can vary from nothing at all, to medications, to a liver transplant, if liver failure occurs. Once diagnosed, a patient will need to have frequent blood test to monitor their condition; a liver biopsy may be obtained every four to eight years as well, to assess the liver. The medications that treat HCV may not be recommended if the patient's liver is in advanced stages of cirrhosis, if they consume alcohol, take IV drugs, have depression, mental illness, are pregnant or might become pregnant, have lupus, rheumatoid arthritis, diabetes, heart disease or seizures.

The treatment will depend on the type of Hepatitis, but could last from a few months to a year. Even if the disease is treated, the infection could still return, as the medication may not permanently get rid of the virus. Side effects of the medication also carry serious risks so it is important to work with your physician to make informed decisions regarding your treatment options. If a liver transplant is necessary, this could entail a long time on the transplant list, and

HOSPITAL INFECTIOUS DISEASES

many patients may die while waiting for a new liver.

Prevention

Prevention can be obtained by some very basic infection control practices. Equipment that comes in contact with blood should never be reused and the area around it should also be sanitized. Hand washing and wearing gloves are very basic, but does not always happen in a clinical setting. The healthcare providers should be doing this not only to protect themselves, but those that they are taking care of. You need to be alert to your surroundings and don't be afraid of asking questions. During my nursing school clinicals, I watched as a physician dropped an instrument on the floor and then put it inside the comatose patient. I was appalled to say the least, so make sure you are getting clean equipment. President Ronald Regan used to say "trust, but verify". We must be proactive in our health and that includes asking questions, watching what is going on and if something seems out of place, say something....Loudly!

Considerations for Hepatitis B & C:

1. Wash hands
2. Wear gloves and protective clothing when handling blood or taking care of infected patients.
3. Do not share needles, toothbrushes, razors or anything that has come in contact with someone else's blood.
4. Make sure your healthcare providers only use sterilized instruments, if they are going "inside" of your body.
5. Keep all cuts or lesions covered and protected.
6. Have protected sex, by using condoms.
7. Talk with your physician to see if you are a candidate to receive the Hepatitis B vaccine.
8. If diagnosed with hepatitis, avoid alcohol and check with your physician before taking new medications as this could damage your liver.

Vancomycin Resistant Enterococci (VRE)

Organisms can change or even undergo random genetic mutations, but the Enterococci changes have made a superbug, resistant to our strongest antibiotics. Vancomycin Resistant Enterococci (VRE) is another bacteria that is typically found in the hospital or physician office settings, but countries outside of the United States have also reported VRE cases outside of healthcare facilities. Officials began to take notice of VRE in the 1980s, and today, it is one of the most common hospital-acquired infections. Many physicians will use Vancomycin as their last alternative for treatment of certain infections, so if Vancomycin cannot be used to treat a patient, there may not be many other choices left. Enterococci are normally found in the intestines, female genital and the environment, but the development of this strain has cost many patients their life.

The CDC reports the number of cases resistant to Vancomycin have almost doubled between 1995 and 2004. They also report that about 30 percent of all enterococci infections were resistant to Vancomycin. Remember that we can live with enterococci bacteria and not have any illness, but when the bacteria colonize, we develop an infection. VRE can also transmit its resistant genes to other more dangerous bacteria and could even put healthy people at risk. If a patient has a weakened immune system and contract VRE, the infection could be a serious threat to their health.

The bacteria can cause an infection anywhere in the body, but it most commonly occurs in the intestines, urinary tract and wounds. Anyone can become infected with the bacteria by contact with individuals that have VRE, after touching a contaminated surface, or by eating contaminated food. VRE can also be found on beds, hospital equipment, doorknobs and hospital personnel.

Hospital personnel and those that cohabitate with VRE patients are at a higher risk of being carriers of the disease without any symptoms. Some European studies estimate that 3.5-5 percent of the total population could be VRE carriers, and could easily pass the infection on to others even though symptoms may not be present.

The older population with a compromised immune system is also at a greater risk for developing this condition. Those most at risk are usually hospitalized patients with illnesses like cancer, immune deficiencies, kidney disease and blood disorders, but no one is exempt. Patients that have had surgery, long-term internal medical devices, or previous Vancomycin treatments are at a greater risk for developing VRE.

Symptoms

Signs and symptoms of VRE depend on the infection location. Most VRE infections will present with a fever, chills, weak feeling and diarrhea. Infected wounds could be red, warm to touch, painful, swelling and may have drainage from the site. Urinary tract and wound infections with VRE can have typical infection symptoms, but no matter where the infection is, a culture will need to be obtained to confirm the diagnosis.

Treatment

Treatment will include a private room to lessen the risk of spreading the infection. The healthcare workers should wear protective clothing such as gloves and gowns. Usually a combination of medications is administered, to attempt control of the bacteria, since it is resistant to so many antibiotics. The physician will continue to monitor the patient's symptoms as well as lab samples taken from the infection location to assess their response to the treatment. Antibiotics may need to be changed if the infection is not responding to the selected treatment regiment.

Wounds with VRE may need to have the fluid drained from the area to relieve the pain and aid in infection reduction. Some patients require that the wound be left "open" after the infection has been drained, to allow for uninhibited drainage. If the wound is left open, with healing, closure of the wound will also take place. Protective sterile dressings should be utilized to protect the patient from other contaminates during this process.

Sometimes patients can fight VRE on their own as their bodies recover and get stronger. How long the patient will be sick depends how the body responds, but it could take months for patients to get rid of this infection. The physician should also be monitoring the patient's intake, as maintaining a proper diet will also assist the body in fighting the war against VRE.

Prevention

Contact precautions need to be implemented with VRE, which means all caregivers should wear a mask, gloves, and gown when taking care of these patients. The patient may be in a private room or with someone that also has VRE depending on the hospital's policies.

VRE can be killed by washing your hands with soap and warm water or even using the alcohol-base hand sanitizers that are often provided in the patient rooms. This practice can also prevent you from becoming a carrier. All wounds or cuts should be protected with a bandage to avoid exposure. Avoid coming in contact with affect substances such as urine, stool and wounds, but wear protective clothing when there could be a possible exposure.

VRE can also live on surfaces such as telephones and stethoscopes for up to 7 days. Health care practitioners should leave necessary equipment, such as blood pressure cuffs, stethoscopes, thermometers in the patient's room, so not to spread the infection on to other patients or visitors.

Find ways to reduce your exposure to potentially contaminated surfaces or objects, and washing items that might have been touched with an infected patient will also reduce the risk of spreading this bacteria. Decrease the use of antibiotics, unless necessary, to reduce the risk for developing resistance to often necessary treatments.

VRE considerations:

1. Wash hands- this can kill the bacteria.
2. Make sure all healthcare providers wash their hands before they see you.
3. Avoid hospitals unless necessary.
4. Clean the environment of patients diagnosed with VRE frequently.
5. Avoid antibiotics unless necessary.

6. Wear protective clothing when visiting someone with VRE.
7. Avoid touching items that could be contaminated.
8. Ask how many cases of VRE your hospital has reported.
9. Avoid eating foods with your hands while at the hospital.
10. Health care providers need to wash their hands, and then put on gloves, prior to touching your food.

Escherichia Coli (E. coli)

E.coli outbreaks have occurred all across the United States from certain food sources, as consuming contaminated food is the most common way to become infected, with this bacteria. This bug knows no limits, as it has warranted multi-million dollar recalls from our food chain. Usually an outbreak can be traced back to one location, but the exact food source may not always be discovered. This condition not only causes undue stress to the patient, but the Centers for Disease Control estimates that $405 million could be spent on E.coli related illnesses each year.

There is one strain of E.coli that has even made it to the bioterrorism list of potential substances. Contamination of our food or water sources has the potential to affect millions of people. Although E. coli can be found in the intestines, some strains can cause violent symptoms. Cattle can also carry the bacteria in their intestines and can be transmitted to the meat during the slaughtering process. Most E.coli outbreaks occur in ground beef, as it can be spread throughout the product during the mixing process. With the E.coli now in the "middle" of the hamburger, it may not be totally "killed" during the cooking process. Those that have "pink" in their hamburger after cooking are at greatest risk for contracting the disease. E-Coli have also been found in contaminated food, water and unpasteurized milk.

The bacteria can be found in our environment, but the strain E. coli O157:H7 has been the culprit in the news lately resulting in hamburger and apple juice recalls. To become infected, all it takes is for an individual to put something in their mouth that has been contaminated with the bacteria, and unfortunately this occurs more than we would like to acknowledge. People have been infected after drinking lake water, unpasteurized apple cider, by eating undercooked meat and contaminated lettuce. Nothing is exempt when it comes to E. coli, not even the local petting zoo, or the public restroom.

The number of persons affected varies from one outbreak to another. The outbreak related to spinach in 2006 left 205 sick and three dead. The Food and Drug Administration (FDA) attempts to keep bacteria from our food chain, but nothing is fool proof, and most often we do not know when something is contaminated until it is too late.

Some patients with E.coli can develop a complication called hemolytic uremic syndrome (HUS). In HUS, the red blood cells are destroyed, which can result in kidney failure. Young children and the elderly are most susceptible to this condition, but anyone can be affected. Many times those with E.coli will end up at the hospital for treatment and potentially could expose others to this bacteria.

Symptoms

E. coli can lead to damage of the intestinal lining which results in severe cramps, diarrhea, nausea and fatigue. The diarrhea can be watery at first and then become bloody. The patient may also have a low-grade fever, nausea and vomiting, which can potentiate dehydration without proper treatment. The symptoms can develop in two to five days after ingestion of the contaminated product, and could continue for up to 8-10 days. Some individuals with E.coli can be infected without any symptom, which increases the risk of the disease spreading. The infection carries some of the same symptoms as other conditions so it is always wise to seek medical attention when abnormal diarrhea symptoms develop, where a culture of the stool can be performed to confirm the diagnosis. Children are also at a greater risk for complications as they can become dehydrated much faster than adults.

Treatment

One of the biggest issues we see in patients with E.coli is dehydration caused by the diarrhea and possible vomiting. If the patient develops more serious problems like anemia or kidney failure, they may be required to have a blood transfusion, dialysis and careful regulation of their fluids and minerals.

Medications are not usually used to treat E.coli and certainly not antidiarrheal products as they will slow down the bacteria leaving the body, increasing the risk of the bacteria affecting the blood and kidneys. Because the symptoms are similar to other intestinal "bugs", the individual with E.coli may take over the counter mediations unknowingly, to treat the diarrhea, but it could result in serious problems. For those that survive their E.coli infection, it usually takes between five and ten days for the symptoms to resolve.

Those that develop serious complications from the E.coli can have life long complications, including paralysis, high blood pressure, seizures or blindness. An E.coli infection could even require the removal of a section of the patient's intestines, which presents its own set of complications and risk factors.

Prevention

Washing your hands could prevent exposure as well as cooking all meat to at least 160 degrees Fahrenheit (internal temperature). Make sure that there is no pink (under cooked) in the hamburger, and consume only pasteurized juices and milks. Do not cross contaminate utensils with raw meat, counter tops or uncooked food. Avoid drinking pond water or even ice from unknown sources. Make sure that you eat your meat while warm to prevent bacteria growth. Proper cleaning of all fresh fruits and vegetables is also necessary to prevent E.coli infection.

Researchers are working on treatments that would aid in the prevention of the disease developing into hemolytic uremic syndrome. Vaccines for both animals and humans are also being researched at this time, but for now, they are not available to the public.

E.coli considerations:
1. Wash hands before eating.
2. Cook meat thoroughly- no pink.
3. Wash hands after using the restroom.
4. Wash all fruits and vegetables.
5. Do not cross contaminate cooking utensils.
6. Contamination could be anywhere at the hospital, so make sure to wash your hands before consuming food or food preparation.
7. Wear gloves when taking care of patients with E.coli.
8. Eating utensils should not come in contact with any possibly contaminated surfaces.

Klebsiella pneumoniae (K. pneumoniae)

K. pneumoniae is a bacteria that has been recognized for over 100 years and is a common hospital acquired pathogen. It accounts for about eight percent of hospital acquired infections in the United States. It can have a mortality rate of almost 50 percent, even with antibiotic treatment. Those with alcoholism or bacteremia can reach almost a 100 percent mortality rate.

It can be found in our intestines, where kept in balance, can keep us healthy. It is commonly found in urinary tract infections or pneumonia, but also can also develop in surgical wounds. K. pneumoniae has been implicated with meningitis, endocarditis and cholangitis as well. It appears that the presence of urinary catheters, contaminated respiratory support equipment and antibiotic use, or over use, are factors that increase the risk of acquiring this infection. Many of these devices utilized in the hospital are there to help the patient get better, but the IV's or urinary tract catheters along with breathing tubes can allow bacteria to get around the body's natural defenses.

A weakened immune system, diseases such as diabetes, alcoholism and chronic lung disease are also considered risk factors. Although most cases are contracted in the hospital, there have been clinical observations of K. *pneumonia* in the community setting that have caused meningitis and liver abscesses. The over use of broad-spectrum antibiotics has led to a strain of the bacteria that are also multi-drug resistant, and these virulent strains have an unbelievable ability to spread, which can result in sepsis or even death.

Symptoms

Those with K. *pneumoniae* of the respiratory tract will generally develop a high fever, flu-like symptoms, and a cough with mucous produced. The mucous can often be thick and tinged with blood. The bacteria can cause lung destruction, inflammation and hemorrhage producing the blood tainted mucus that looks like currant jelly. Pockets of pus or abscesses can form and may also result in a surgical procedure to remove them. The pus can also surround the lung and cause irritation which results in scarring. Symptoms of urinary tract infections (UTI) with a catheter do not usually have the "normal" signs and symptoms of a UTI, as a catheter is generally in place, so the urine is flowing freely, which can lessen the normal UTI symptoms. It is also possible that the urine will have a cloudy appearance in the catheter bag or those without a catheter can experience incontinence, urinary frequency, fever, flank pain and confusion. Sometimes it will be the blood work that grabs the physician's attention with an elevated white cell count as the catheter induced urinary tract infections can even be asymptomatic. Surgical wounds can present with typical symptoms of infection including redness, tenderness, fever and drainage from the wound site.

Treatment

The diagnosis is obtained through a culture of the infected area usually requiring either a sputum, blood or urine sample. X-rays can also be obtained to assess the lung condition for respiratory infections. For surgical wounds, a swab of the affected area will be collected, and sent to the lab. The lab will determine which antibiotics the bacteria are sensitive to, so the physician will order the "right" treatment regiment. These cultures can take two to three days, but the doctor might not wait for the results before initiating antibiotics.

Physicians will often prescribe a "hard hitting" antibiotic until they know the lab results and then change if necessary once the results are in. The antibiotic regiment could last 10-14 days depending on the location and how the patient responds to the treatment. Some infections could take weeks of antibiotic therapy, and may require more than one antibiotic at a time. Bandages with silver in them have also been beneficial with surgical wound healing, as the silver acts as an antimicrobial.

Prevention

This is a condition that is generally found in the hospital so the best thing to do for prevention is try to stay healthy. Reduce your risk factors by limiting your alcohol intake, get proper rest and eat a healthy diet.

If you are a patient that needs certain medical devices, make sure that the only tubes (IV's, breathing equipment and catheters) used are absolutely necessary. If the devices are required, make sure that they are removed as soon as possible. Avoid being in close proximity to patients with pneumonia or coming in contact with infected mucus, urine or wounds. Wear a mask and gloves, and then wash hands after handling contaminated objects. If you know that your immune system is compromised, stay away from the hospital, or those that are ill.

K. pneumoniae considerations:

1. Wash hands meticulously to prevent contracting or spreading this bacteria.
2. Maintain a healthy lifestyle and monitor chronic diseases such as diabetes.
3. Avoid those that are ill if your immune system is compromised.
4. Medical devices should be sterile prior to insertion.
5. All internal medial devices should be removed as soon as your condition allows.
6. Assess the hospital's and physician's infection rate, prior to any surgical procedures.

7. Wear gloves, gowns and masks (if respiratory) when caring for, or visiting infected patients.
8. Avoid alcohol consumption to lower the risk of contracting this pathogen.

Tuberculosis (TB)

TB is a bacteria called Mycobacterium tuberculosis, and has been around for many years. This condition usually attacks the lungs, but has been found to affect the kidneys, spine and brain. It can be a fatal disease if not treated properly and the CDC reports in the past, this disease was once the leading cause of death in the United States. The infection has been on the decline since 1993 but still continues to be a problem today. TB asylums were a very common place in most communities not that long ago, but it is better managed today with the antibiotics available to us.

Some of the bacteria can live inside of our bodies like many others without causing us any harm. If these atypical mycobacteria do cause an infection, it can present symptoms like TB. The atypical condition is different than the active type, so the drug treatment could last for one to two years with multiple medications.

It is an airborne bacteria that can cause respiratory symptoms, but some people infected with the bacteria may not have any symptoms, yet are still contagious. The tiny bacteria infect a person after inhalation of the particles from the sputum. The bacteria can be spread in the air just by someone coughing, sneezing, shouting or spitting. Individuals cannot become infected by touching clothes or the belongings of someone infected with TB, but can be expose just by inhaling the bacteria.

The atypical form of TB has also been transmitted by drinking unpasteurized milk, but rarely occurs now that most milk is pasteurized. Here in Michigan, we have seen cases of TB in deer, elk, black bear, raccoon, fox, bobcats, opossum, and coyote. The

Michigan DNR has reported that as few as 42 percent of the TB positive white-tail deer have had lesions in the chest or lungs and encourage the hunters to perform an extensive assessment of the deer's lymph nodes to prevent the consumption of contaminated meat.

The United States reports an average of 22,000 new cases each year, but believes that 10-15 million people are infected at this time. It is much more prevalent in other parts of the world with as many as eight million new cases reported each year. With the emergence of immune compromised HIV patients, TB has remained a public concern. Those at highest risk are individuals that live with patients that have active TB, the poor or homeless, alcoholics, intravenous drug users, those with weakened immune systems, diabetes or cancer.

Health care workers are also at high risk due to caring for patients prior to a confirmed diagnosis. Those living or visiting countries with high TB rates are also at risk for exposure to this condition. Individuals living in nursing homes or prisons have a higher prevalence, and certain medical treatments like steroids or rheumatoid arthritis medications can put you at risk if you are exposed to TB.

Symptoms

The latent TB infection can lay dormant for years without causing any symptoms, but when the immune system cannot fight the bacteria off, symptoms will develop. Patients with TB report weakness or fatigue, weight loss, loss of appetite, fever and night sweats. The progression of the disease can result in symptoms of coughing, chest pain, coughing up mucus (with or without blood) and shortness of breath. If the bacteria go beyond the lungs, the symptoms will vary depending on the organs affected. See Graph 5 for the comparison of Latent TB vs. Active TB.

HOSPITAL INFECTIOUS DISEASES

A person with Latent TB Infection	A person with Active TB
• Does not feel sick	• Usually feels sick
• Has no symptoms	Symptoms may include: -A bad cough, pain in the chest, coughing up blood or sputum, weight loss, loss of appetite, chills, fever and night sweats.
• Usually has a positive skin test or positive TB blood test	• Usually has a positive skin test or positive TB blood test
• Cannot spread TB bacteria to others	• Is contagious to others.
• Treatment should be considered to prevent active TB disease later.	• Does not need treatment
• Has a negative sputum smear, and a normal chest x-ray.	• May have a positive sputum smear or culture, or an abnormal chest x-ray.

A skin test will be done if TB is suspected, but a positive TB skin test means that you have been exposed to the disease, but a false negative can occur if the exposure has occurred recently. It can take 2-10 weeks after exposure for the TB skin test to result as positive. For those with weakened immune systems due to conditions like AIDS or cancer, the test can also show a false-negative. Once the skin test is positive, a chest X-ray and possibly a sputum culture will be obtained to evaluate the stage of the disease. The chest X-ray can show active and inactive TB while the analysis of the sputum can tell the physician if the disease is TB or atypical TB, but this can take up to six weeks in the laboratory before results are generated. There is a test that analyzes a short sequence of DNA that could provide your physician with results in just a few days.

Treatment
The treatment regiment for TB varies, depending on if the TB

is active or latent. If the patient has the inactive condition (latent), the physician will most likely recommend an antibiotic regiment to prevent the bacteria from becoming active. The drug of choice is isoniazid (INH) and is usually prescribed for 6-12 months. Even with this treatment, the patient still carries up to a 10 percent change of developing an active TB infection. There are cases where the antibiotic treatment is not recommended, so make sure to understand all of the risks associated with taking this medication.

If the patient has a positive TB test, abnormal chest X-ray and sputum, the TB is contagious and should be treated with a combination of medications including isoniazid, rifampin, ethambutol and pyrazinamide. Usually all four medications are taken for the first two months, then only two medications for the rest of the time, depending on drug sensitivity to the bacteria. Medication can be administered for months to even years and the successfulness of the treatment usually depends on the patient's compliance with the recommended regiment. If the medication treatment fails, surgery may be necessary on the lungs, but this is typically not the case. Early detection and treatment regiment can assist with a successful recovery for the patient.

Prevention

Visitors or caregivers of active TB patients must wear a special type of mask called N95, which does not let the tiny TB particles into the respiratory tract. A generic paper mask will not prevent the inhalation of the TB bacteria. The patient with active TB will be put in an isolation room with specialize ventilation not to spread the infected particles throughout the hospital.

It will take two to three days to get the results of the skin test, so it might be worth waiting for the diagnosis before visiting someone with suspected TB, but remember there is also a chance of a false-negative. If you know that you have been around someone with TB, see your doctor right away. There is a vaccine against TB, but is usually not administered in the United States. The vaccinated person will generally show a false-positive after the vaccination which also

HOSPITAL INFECTIOUS DISEASES

causes confusion when trying to diagnosis the disease. Because we cannot physically see TB, we do not often know when we have been exposed. A friend of mine worked with under-privileged children, and had a positive TB skin test at her annual physical, but she had no idea when she had been exposed.

Healthcare workers are also required to take annual TB test to assess for exposure, and if you work in high risk areas, you too should be tested. Many people report symptoms for several weeks before they seek medical attention so definitely be aware of those people coughing around you.

Considerations for TB
1. Know your risks for TB exposure and report any possible exposure immediately to your physician.
2. TB symptoms require immediate medical attention to avoid spreading the disease as well as prompt treatment for your condition.
3. Wear N95 masks when around patients with active TB.
4. Those with a weakened immune system or chronic disease, should avoid exposure to people with active TB, or visiting areas with a high incidence of TB.
5. Health care providers or those living with TB patients should have a TB skin test annually.
6. Complete the TB treatment regiment as prescribed for the entire duration.

Pseudomonas aeruginosa (P. aeruginosa)

P. aeruginosa is a bacteria that usually lives in the soil and water, but can also live on plants and animals. It doesn't usually cause disease in a healthy person, but for those with weakened immune systems it can be deadly. Most patients in the hospital have some form of a compromised immune system or they probably would not be there. The bacteria gained a little more notoriety in 2009 after a Brazilian beauty queen developed a urinary tract infection that went to her blood stream, which resulted in the amputation of her hands and feet, and eventually took her life. Although this is uncommon in healthy individuals, we must recognize the dangers that we all face.

According to the CDC, around 10 percent of the two million nosocomial infections that occur each year are caused by P. aeruginosa. Infection caused by this bacteria can develop in the urinary tract, respiratory system, intestinal tract, soft tissue, bone, joints, skin, and the blood. This bacteria is the 2nd leading cause of all hospital acquired pneumonias and the leading cause of pneumonias and urinary tract infections in the ICU.

It is usually found in water sources, including hospital sinks, but can also be found in birthing tubs, swimming pools, hot tubs and whirlpools as it thrives in the warm temperatures. Patients with cystic fibrosis, cancer and burns carry the highest fatality rate near 50 percent. Because this bacteria thrives in oxygen rich environments, it can live on basic hospital equipment like oxygen masks, breathing apparatuses or urinary catheters despite cleaning.

Swimmer's ear can be caused by P.aeruginosa which can be a minor infection, but could possibly lead to ear infections which result in hearing loss, facial paralysis or even death in elderly patients. Studies have found different modes of transmission in the hospital setting for the bacteria, but one hospital reported that 16 babies had died from this infection over a 15 month period, and found that nurses wearing artificial nails were the carriers. Other infections have occurred when instruments used to insert breathing tubes had not been sterilized properly and also resulted in death. Healthcare providers can carry the bacteria on their hands or stethoscopes which can put those with compromised immune systems at risk for developing the infection.

Water is used throughout the hospital setting for a variety of reasons, so it is not surprising infections have developed after water baths were used to warm dialysis fluids, fresh-frozen plasma and albumin. Bathing premature infants has also been discouraged as the water can expose the baby's immature immune system to these dangerous bacteria.

Symptoms

The symptoms vary according to the location of the infection. For endocarditis, the patient may have a fever, heart murmur and positive blood cultures. Pneumonia patients can have fever, a blue tint to the skin, decreased oxygen saturation and difficulty breathing.

Gastrointestinal tract infections are generally seen in infants and can produce symptoms of diarrhea, fever, dehydration and an enlarged abdomen. Infections of the skin and soft tissues vary from a rash to hemorrhagic or necrotic tissue. Patients with burns can quickly have an infection that spreads throughout the body and may have symptoms of disorientation, low blood pressure, decreased urine output, low body temperature, bowel obstruction and a decrease of white blood cells. If the infection is located in the blood, the patient can experience fever, rapid heart, increased respirations, jaundice, decreased blood pressure and skin lesions.

Treatment

Treatment of P. *aeruginosa* can be difficult as the bacteria have become resistant to many of our antibiotics. It usually requires a combination of multiple antibiotics for two to six weeks to treat this infection. If the infection is in the eye, antibiotic eye drops are usually required. Burn units often require irrigation therapy and should use a "clean" water source and decontaminate tubing between uses to lessen the exposure to P. aeruginosa. Surgery may be necessary if the tissue has been damaged, and could even require amputation of limbs if the damage is permanent. Treatment is generally successful but patients with infections of the heart can have an 89 percent mortality rate according to the Visiting Nurses Association research.

Prevention

Maintain your health and stay out of compromised situations. The less you are in the hospital; the less you are exposed to the bacteria. Make sure the hospital has prevention methods in place which should include cleaning of the water system. Those with cystic fibrosis should be provided antibiotics regularly as a preventative

SURVIVING YOUR MEDICAL CRISIS

measure. Avoid IV or urinary catheterizations, and request that the medical device be removed as soon as possible if you do require a catheter. The catheter should also be inserted under sterile conditions, and if you do require long term catheterization, it should be replaced frequently, to reduce the risk for P. *aeruginosa* infections. All of the healthcare providers should wash their hands prior to any contact or treatments, and wear gloves accordingly. Patients should also wash their hands to reduce exposure or further spreading of the infection.

Avoid public swimming pools and hot tubs with cloudy water. Make sure that the birthing tubs have been thoroughly disinfected and you weigh the risk of potential contamination still being in the tubs. When it comes to cleaning anything at the hospital, I like to compare it to getting your car washed. The water is always coming down so hard, the brushes are scrubbing every inch, and soap covers the whole car. After washing, the car gets blown away by the dryers, and there are people that dry it off with towels, and yet, there can still be dirt left on the car. Your health is so much more important than your car, so ask questions, weigh the risk and make informed decisions.

P. *aeruginosa* considerations:
1. Maintain a healthy lifestyle.
2. Those with a compromised immune system, should stay away from the hospital unless necessary.
3. Make sure your healthcare providers are not wearing artificial nails.
4. Take preventative antibiotics if you have cystic fibrosis.
5. Make sure the healthcare providers wash their hands and clean their equipment prior to touching you or initiating treatment.
6. Avoid public swimming pools and hot tubs with cloudy water.
7. Make sure the hospital equipment is sterilized properly before treatment initiation.

Acinetobacter baumannii (A baumannii)

This is not a new bacteria as it can be found in our environment, including the soil, vegetables, meat, fish and our skin. It can live on dry surfaces like; skin, equipment or contaminated surfaces for up to 20 days. For the average person, this bacteria may not be of much concern, but for patients in the hospital, or those that have a compromised immune system, precautions will need to be taken. A. baumannii has not got as much publicity as other super-bugs, because it doesn't usually kill healthy people, but this bacteria is resistant to multiple drugs, and has 52 genes that are solely responsible for defeating antibiotics or radiation.

The bacteria was reported in our wounded troops in Iraq around 2003, and has since been found at our military hospital in Germany and at Walter Reed, here in the states. It has been reported that over 700 military deaths have occurred from this bacteria. In 2005 we saw outbreaks in various cities across the United States with around 97 percent of the cases all coming from one strain or originating from one source. A. baumannii has the great ability to mutate rapidly and the unrestricted use of antibiotics has aided the emergence of this super strain.

It was not until 2007 that the military and the civilian world started sharing their information on the bacterial infection statistics. Hospitals here in the United States do not have to report infections caused by this bacteria, so actual cases of this condition may be hard to confirm.

The infections caused by A. baumannii are generally seen in critically ill patients, the elderly, major trauma or burn patients. With these patients we usually see indwelling catheters, long hospital stays, antibiotic administration and mechanical ventilation, which all put the patient at higher risk for infection. The bacteria usually cause infections of the skin, soft tissue, respiratory tract, urinary tract, peritoneal cavity, blood and even secondary meningitis. Pneumonia and wound infections have also been contracted in the community setting in other countries, but those with chronic diseases like diabetes, COPD, renal failure, tobacco or alcohol consumption are at greatest risk.

Symptoms

Symptoms vary with the location of the infection. In pneumonia cases, symptoms could include a cough, fever and chills, but the bacteria have also been found in wounds or tracheostomy sites without any symptoms present. Fever, pain, foul drainage and redness around the infected wounds can be reported. Common symptoms of urinary tract infections like fever, flank pain or painful urination can also occur, but are not necessary for the infection to be present.

Rare cases of meningitis caused by this bacteria, can have a fever, headache, stiff neck, dislike for bright lights and mental status changes. Blood infection symptoms will usually have a fever, chills and general "ill feeling", while elevated white cell counts can be an indication of infection anywhere.

Treatment

There are very few antibiotics that effectively treat A. baumannii, but the multi-resistant strain leaves few to choose from. These gold-standard antibiotics are often the ones used as a last resort, with serious side affects, and need to be taken with a full understanding of what side effects could be experienced. Side effects could include stomach upset, diarrhea, a rash, hearing loss, impaired liver or kidney function. For those patients that may have the bacteria on their skin or wounds without any infection, no antibiotics are usually prescribed, but can be administered in these "carrier" patients if there is concern for transmission or infection is a high possibility.

Prevention

Because most patients are exposed to this in the healthcare setting, it is important to pay attention to the environment, and also make sure that all healthcare providers wash their hands thoroughly. The tables and sinks need to also be sanitized every day, and every item taken to the hospital needs to be cleaned with a disinfectant or washed. The bacteria can live on surfaces for several days, so infection control practices need to be implemented by all healthcare providers for the risk of contracting A. baumannii to be reduced.

Prevention considerations:
1. Lower your risk of needing hospital services, including outpatient surgery.
2. Avoid touching the skin of infected or colonized individuals.
3. Wash your hands frequently if you have the infection or if you visit someone with this condition.
4. All healthcare providers must wash their hands and instruments prior to contact.
5. Only use antibiotics when absolutely necessary.
6. Bring only necessary things into the hospital room.
7. All dressings need to be secure and inform the nurse if they are loose or wet.
8. Keep IV dressing intact.
9. Make sure chronic conditions like diabetes is under control.

Human Immunodeficiency Virus (HIV and AIDS)

HIV is a retrovirus that causes acquired immunodeficiency syndrome (AIDS) in the later stages of the disease. We all know that our immune system plays such an important part in our health, but when a patient develops AIDS, their immune system begins to fail and they are left to face opportunistic viruses and infections or cancers alone. Patients can live for many years before the condition develops into AIDS, as new anti-viral treatments are being developed and research for a cure continues. Once a patient's condition develops into AIDS, it more than likely will result in AIDS-related illnesses, which could take their life.

The World Health Organization (WHO) estimated that 33.2 million people worldwide had HIV by 2007, with 2.5 million of those being new diagnosis. They also estimated that around 2.1 million people died of AIDS in 2007. The CDC estimates that there were 56,300 new cases of HIV in the United States in 2006, and noted that there was a 15 percent increase from 2004-2007 in the 34 states that report this disease.

Anyone can be infected with the disease through sexual transmission, infected blood, sharing of needles or needle sticks, and from their mother if she was HIV positive during pregnancy. There have also been reports of the virus being transmitted through organ donations and unsterilized dental or surgical equipment. Though rare, there have even been reports of transmission from an infected dentist to six of his patients.

Most patients are diagnosed by a blood test, and can be performed anonymously, but there is an alternative saliva test that is very accurate. Although most studies say that HIV cannot be transmitted through the saliva, there are HIV antibodies present in saliva of HIV positive patients.

Symptoms

HIV is a progressive disease that will end up with full blown AIDS. In the beginning, HIV could have symptoms similar to the flu, like nausea, vomiting, diarrhea, fever, enlarged lymph nodes, headache, weight loss, sore throat, rash, general aches and pains. They vary in the severity, but usually disappear after two to three weeks. Many do not even know that they have been infected at this stage and it may take years for the HIV symptoms to fully develop.

In the mean time, the virus is multiplying in their body, even if they do not have any symptoms. It may not be until they have unexplained symptoms like confusion, dry cough, mouth sores, night sweats, numbness in extremities or yeast infections (to name a few) that an HIV diagnoses will be given. HIV may be suspected in children if they have an enlarged spleen or delayed growth. Once AIDS develops, which could take 12-13 years if untreated, the immune system is rendered weakened and other infections like pneumonia or cancer take advantage of the body's weakened state. There is a small chance of a rapid progression of the disease which could develop into AIDS within three years, but this is not as common in the United States.

Treatments

There are several antiretroviral medications on the market, as well as immune system boosters that can assist in deferring the disease. There is no cure at this present time for HIV/AIDS. It appears that once the virus gets a foothold in the body, it cannot be eradicated. There are many people that are effectively "living" with the disease by taking antiviral drugs and immune boosters. Patients with HIV must work closely with their healthcare provider when evaluating treatment methods as the medications carry multiple side effects including toxicity and resistance to the HIV drugs.

Prevention

HIV does not survive well outside of the body so the preventative measures focuses on your behavior. Do not have any sexual contact (oral, anal or vaginal) unless you know the person is free of HIV, and if you do have sex, make sure to use condoms to assist with prevention of sexually transmitted diseases.

Get tested if you practice high risk behaviors such as multiple partners, homosexual relations, and illicit drug use, or have been diagnosed with another sexually transmitted disease like gonorrhea, syphilis or chlamydia trachomatis as these can all increase your risk of getting HIV.

You also need to inform those around if you have HIV/AIDS, especially your sexual partners or people that you share needles with. This may not be an easy task, but you could be putting their life at risk by not telling them. Healthcare providers or individuals that may come in contact with your blood should also be made aware for their protection. Charges have been brought against HIV/AIDS patients that have not disclosed their health status to their partners, and transmitted the disease. Full disclosure is best, as this allows the partner to make informed decisions.

Considerations for HIV/AIDS

1. Protect yourself by avoiding contact with infected blood.
2. Do not share needles.
3. Have protected sex.

4. Get tested if you are at risk.
5. HIV does not live outside of the body so the environment is of low concern.
6. Take necessary precautions like gloves, facemasks and covering of your wounds when there is a possibility of exposed to an infected person's blood.
7. Inform any sexual partner or healthcare providers of your health status.
8. Do not donate blood if you are HIV/AIDS positive.

Aspergillus fungus

There has been a dramatic increase of the disease aspergillosis which is caused by the Aspergillus fungus over the last few decades, even with improved diagnostic, and treatment efforts. This fungus forms spores and is generally found in our environment, including soil, water, food, dust and plants. Hospital ventilation systems are also a habitat for the spores, which can be transmitted in the air during construction or renovation projects. Reports have indicated that the spores can also come from wet wood, eroding fireproofing materials or through bird droppings near the hospital air ducts.

Illness from the spores can range from allergy-type reactions to life threatening situations. Community-acquired infections can occur as it is almost impossible for people to totally avoid breathing spores from the environment. *Aspergillus* can cause infection in the bronchi and the lungs although infections of the skin have also been reported after contact with contaminated biomedical devices. Those with highest susceptibility are bone marrow, organ or stem cell recipients, as well as cancer patients. Patients with conditions like diabetes, major burns, alcoholism, major surgery or corticosteroids use, all have a potentially higher risk for becoming infected with this fungus.

Pneumonia is often the most serious result of spore inhalation with outbreaks occurring most often in intensive care units in patients with respiratory conditions or bone marrow transplants. The spores can also result in sinusitis and can disseminate to other places in the body. Those with asthma or cystic fibrosis may also find this fungus to be very difficult to deal with.

John Hopkins reports that the mortality of patients with pneumonia caused by Aspergillus could be as high as 85 percent. That is an alarming percentage considering that 12.5 percent of high risk patients could develop this infection. Outbreaks occur usually when air duct systems become contaminated, but some hospitals have implemented better ventilation systems and have seen a reduction of this infection. If Aspergillosis is not treated, it could lead to permanent lung damage, respiratory failure, or airway obstruction.

The condition can be diagnosed with an Aspergillus antigen skin test, bronchoscopy biopsy, chest X-ray, CT of the chest and specialized blood tests. A sputum sample can also be tested for the fungus, and with a proper diagnosis and treatment the patient can begin the recovery process.

Symptoms

With the respiratory system being the main focus of the infection, patients usually experience fever, chest pain, coughing and spitting up blood. Mild symptoms can vary from the patient just not feeling well, to coughing, wheezing or asthma like symptoms. When Aspergillosis develops in the lungs we can see small fibrous balls, consisting of blood clots, fungus and white blood cells. If these balls enlarge, lung destruction can occur. The condition can spread rapidly throughout the body in patients with weakened immune systems as it travels through the blood stream, and death could come quite quickly. Those with an allergic type of reaction can experience chronic coughing, wheezing and fever. Cultures are reviewed to identify the presence of the fungus, but an X-ray or CT of the infected area may also indicate the presence of the condition.

Treatment

Patients with a serious infection will require antifungal drugs. There are a few medications available for treatment, but it may be necessary to change the antifungal medications if the patient does not respond to the treatment. Corticosteroids can also be administered to reduce the patient's hypersensitive reaction to the spores. Asthma patients will usually stay on their regular medications as well.

Those with mild infections could successfully get rid of the condition by scraping out the fungus or applying topical antifungal drugs for skin reactions. Surgery may be necessary for patients with sinus or lung infections caused by Aspergillus fungus.

Considerations for Aspergillus fungus:
1. Find out if your hospital has HEPA filtration on their ventilation system. This is especially important if construction or renovation work is going on around the building.
2. If your immune system is compromised in any way, stay away from the hospital and environments where fungus could be present.
3. Avoid working in or around compost piles, decaying leaves, wood or plants.
4. Wear N95 masks if working in dusty environments.
5. Make sure that all medical devices are sterilized properly.

Isolation

There are many conditions or diseases that can put patients in an isolation status. Sometimes it will be to protect you from being exposed to other sick patients, while other times it will be utilized to protect the patients from you. Many hospitals today have private patient rooms, so the patient can be in "isolation" in a normal room. On units with multi-patient rooms, there are individual rooms that are designated for isolation. Some hospitals use the same rooms for patients with infectious diseases as they do for those that need to be protected from diseases. The rooms are just cleaned in between each patient. It is important to know how thoroughly a hospital cleans their rooms. Some of the websites report on hospital cleanliness, so this takes on a whole new meaning when the patient needs to be protected from "hospital bugs". Make sure that the room has been

HOSPITAL INFECTIOUS DISEASES

disinfected properly, and notify the manager if the room does not appear to be clean. Be proactive as your health can depend on the housekeeper!

Each hospital is set up differently for isolation rooms, so it is necessary to find out how or where the isolation rooms are managed. Our daughter visited a friend that was in "isolation", but the only indicator was a small sign on the door that she walked right by. She had been exposed and did not even know it. You need to be informed of the patient's condition and what your risks are for exposure. If visiting, your health status also needs to be considered, not only for your health, but for the patient's health. If you know you are ill, stay away from the hospital, as the patients do not need to have any extra "bugs" lurking around.

For certain conditions, the proper attire (masks, gowns and gloves) need to be available outside the patient's door if the patient is allowed visitors. If no supplies are outside of the door, just ask the nurse for the necessary attire, as sometimes they just get all used up and no one has had the time to replenish the supplies.

Do not take food into isolation rooms as it could become contaminated with contagious pathogens. Remember the illustration of getting your car washed. We will not see the infectious "bugs" but they can be everywhere. The chance of the patient having a "bad bug", or even the patient that was in the room before them, is very high. Even though the room is "clean", everything may not be gone. We do not live in a sterile environment, and the hospital rooms are definitely not. For patients with TB, the isolation rooms require special ventilation and these may be only found only on certain units.

Isolation Considerations:
1. Wash Hands, Wash Hands, Wash Hands.
2. Wear protective clothing when applicable.
3. Understand what type of isolation you or the patient is in.
4. Understand there is always a possibility that the patient has infectious bacteria that has not been identified yet.

5. Do not take food into isolation rooms.
6. Remove your clothing when you get home and wash as appropriate.
7. Maintain your health through proper diet and exercise as directed.
8. New "bugs" can develop all the time, so stay on top of what the patient is being tested for.

CHAPTER 5

Transfusions

Almost 5 million people will need a blood transfusion in the United States this year, and 1 in 10 patients admitted to the hospital will need a transfusion. Although the reasons that a transfusion may be required vary, the results could be life saving. The benefits need to be weighed against the risks associated with a transfusion and it should only be done when absolutely necessary.

Many hospitals will have a patient sign a general consent for blood products when they arrive at the emergency room and it will be effective for their entire hospital visit. Others have consents that are effective either in the emergency room or on the inpatient units. This is one of those times it is important for everyone to "read the fine print" before signing the paperwork, as most people come to the emergency room not feeling well and could overlook something very important.

There are different parts of the blood that may be necessary for treatment, including Red blood cells, Platelets or Plasma. The Red blood cells are the transporters of the oxygen to the tissue and organs, and also take the carbon dioxide back to the lungs. The Platelets are the "sticky" part of the blood with their main function being to stop bleeding. Plasma carries water and nutrients to the body's tissues while the proteins in the plasma also help the blood to clot.

Where the blood comes from

There are two different methods for blood transfusion. A patient can receive a transfusion from their own donated blood (Autologous) or they can receive blood from someone else (Allogeneic). In cases of pre-scheduled surgery, a patient may be able to donate their own blood to have on hand incase a transfusion is necessary. The National Blood Data Resource Center reports that around five percent of the blood donations are autologous. The patient must be medically stable and infection free before this type of donation will be considered. The risk for complication from the patient receiving their own blood is low, but make sure to cover this detail with your physician if you require a transfusion. Only about 56 percent of the blood donated for "self-use" is ever needed for treatment, and current regulations do not generally allow it to be used for someone else.

We often hear the American Red Cross requesting blood donations as they have been great pioneers for this cause and their efforts have saved countless numbers of lives. They are requesting donations that will be used for allogeneic type of transfusions. During emergency or surgical situations a patient may have lost volumes of blood that need to be replaced. Patients going through cancer treatments often experience a temporary time that the bone marrow just does not make enough new blood cells, or a patient may also be experiencing anemia (a lack of red blood cells) due to a medical condition, which may require a transfusion.

If a patient is receiving frequent blood transfusions, they may also be at risk for high iron levels. The total number of transfusions over a patient's lifetime is important as the iron from any transfusion stays in the patient's blood. Surprisingly, a patient can be anemic and still have a high iron level in their blood.

TRANSFUSIONS

Blood Donation

With millions of people requiring blood products each year, donations are needed on a regular basis. The products have a shelf-life of anywhere from five days for Platelets to one year for Fresh Frozen Plasma. The hospitals buy and sell these products to make sure that each one is utilized to the best potential. The basic donator requirements ask that a donor be:
- In generally good health and not feeling ill.
- 17 years old or older
- At least 110 pounds
- Heart rate of 80-100 beats/min
- Temperature not over 99.5
- Blood Pressure between 110/60 to 160/90
- Skin around donation site is free of lesions or previous needle pricks.

Please do not donate blood if:
- You have tested positive for HIV
- You are a man and have had sex with another man, even once.
- You have engaged in sex for drugs or money
- You have lived in western Europe since 1980
- You have been in a correctional facility for more than 72 hours in the last 12 months.
- If you have injected illicit drugs or substances.
- You were born in, lived in or had sex with anyone who lived in, or received blood products in Cameroon, Central African Republic, Chad, Congo, Equatorial, Guinea, Gabon, Niger or Nigeria since 1977.
- You are currently or have been in sexual contact with someone in the above list.
- Special concerns for those who have lived or visited England/United Kingdom from 1980-1999 and those who have lived or worked in Western Europe since 1980.

This is just a short list of considerations, but the collecting organization will have a more detailed screening process.

The Type: A, B, AB and O

Getting the right blood type is one of the most important factors in a transfusion. There are four types of blood: A, B, AB and O. The test done prior to the transfusion should include an antigen test to insure the patient will receive the correct blood product type. Acute Hemolytic Transfusion Reactions (HTR) develops when the patient is transfused with an incompatible blood product. Precautionary measures should be in place at most hospitals, but errors have occurred that have even resulted in the patient's death. Even if the patient has a certain blood type, they may be able to receive another type for a transfusion. The graph below provides that information.

Blood types that match	
A person who has:	Can receive:
A- blood	A-, O- blood
A+ blood	A-, A+, O-, O+ blood
B- blood	B-, O- blood
B+ blood	B-, B+, O-, O+ blood
AB- blood	AB-, O- blood
AB+ blood	AB-, AB+, A-, A+, B-, B+, O-, O+ blood
O- blood	O- blood
O+ blood	O-, O+ blood

Transfusion Risks

Non-infectious Risk

Reactions can be caused by various factors. Sometimes a reaction is caused by the white blood cells, so red blood cell products can have the white cells removed (Leukocyte reduced) to prevent reactions from occurring. There can also be an anaphylaxis type reaction where the exact reason may be unknown, but can be very scary for the patient. This reaction can take place during the transfusion or even hours after it is completed. This type of reaction is serious as it can lead to the patient's death. If you have an HTR there is a 1 in 500,000 chance that it could be fatal. Most fatalities associated with HTRs could be prevented, as it is usually caused by human error.

Transfusion-related acute lung injury reactions usually occur within one to two hours of the transfusion. The lungs quickly fill with fluid causing respiratory difficulties. An estimated 40,000 patients will develop this condition each year. An allergic type reaction can also develop and usually occurs shortly after the transfusion is started. The patient may just be sensitive to the allergens in the blood.

There is also a risk for graft versus host disease where the body cannot destroy the incompatible white blood cells. This occurs frequently in patients with compromised immune systems or in those taking immunosuppressant drugs. The symptoms can develop 8-10 days after the transfusion and can result in death a few weeks later.

Infection Risk

Blood donation regulations have provided a safer blood supply for our patients. Public concerns are generally focused on HIV, Hepatitis and bacterial infections. Other conditions like Cytomegalovirus, Lyme disease, Herpes virus, West Nile virus, Mad Cow disease, Malaria and parasites are of equal concern for the medical community.

The screening process for donors requires detailed information to assess the donor's risk for current or potential infectious diseases. Once the blood is collected, the screening process also analyzes the blood for various infectious disease markers. Patients that received transfusions back in the 1980's contracted HIV before some of these new regulations and screening processes were in place. In 1987 the risk associated for contracting HIV with a transfusion was about 1 in 250,000, but by the year 2000, that risk had gone down to 1 in every 2,135,000 transfusions.

There could be infectious diseases in the donated blood that we are currently not aware of, but precautions implemented today are based on current evidence. The chances of contacted an infectious disease through transfusion are much less than acquiring a nosocomial infection.

What to Expect at Transfusion

Blood products should be checked for compatibility with the patient's blood. The nurse should also double-check all labels and identification numbers to make sure they match the patient's. It is possible that the nurse was provided the blood product, but it has someone else's name on it. There should be a two-nurse check system in place for all blood product verification. The nurse should have proper equipment for each product, and should stay with the patient for the first five to fifteen minutes to assess for reaction. Frequent assessments by the nurse should be conducted while the product is transfusing, which includes monitoring the patient's temperature and blood pressure, and making clinical evaluations of the patient's tolerance of the transfusion.

The patient should stay awake during the transfusion and let the nurse know immediately if they are feeling any symptoms of reaction. Red blood cells are usually transfused over two to three hours as the transfusion need to be complete within four hours. If the transfusion goes over four hours, there is concern of possible bacterial contamination of the product. If the patient's condition requires more than one transfusion, the filter in the tubing should be changed after four hours or sooner if it is impaired by debris. The rate of transfusion varies by the product being transfused and the patient's condition. There are possible complications of kidney failure, anaphylaxis and Congestive Heart Failure from transfusions that are administered too fast.

Signs and Symptoms of Reaction

Reactions to the transfusion can occur anytime and the patient may not know if they will react until the product is transfused.

Although most transfusions take place in the hospital, the adverse affects usually occur either during the transfusion or within 24 hours. The graft verses host reaction could take 8-10 days for symptoms to develop. The most frequent reactions are fever, chills, back pain, skin rash, hives and itching, but the patient can also experience respiratory difficulties, severe headache, chest pain or blood in their urine.

Surgical Risk

Recent studies have indicated that heart bypass patients that receive transfusions during surgery are at greater risk for infections and even dying after the operation. The University of Michigan's Safety Enhancement Program reported that transfused patients were five times more likely to die than non-transfused patients in the first 100 days after surgery. This could explain the higher death rates in women who have bypass surgery, as they tend to receive more blood transfusions. If the patient is able to use their own blood, the rate of infections drops considerably, so ask your physician if you are a candidate for donating your own blood prior to surgery.

Transfusion Considerations:

1. Make sure you understand the risks associated with the transfusion and weigh them against the benefits.
2. You need to give consent for blood transfusions, except in emergency situations where consent is not possible.
3. You can refuse the transfusion, but understand the risk associated with this decision.
4. Let the physician and medical personnel know if you have ever had an allergic reaction to any blood product transfusion.
5. Antihistamines can be administered along with acetaminophen prior to a transfusion to lessen your risk for reaction.
6. Donate your own blood if possible before surgery.
7. Make sure your blood and the blood product are compatible prior to the transfusion.
8. Stay awake during your transfusion to assess for reaction.
9. Notify the nurse immediately if any reaction symptoms develop.

CHAPTER 6

The ICU and Your Medical Plan

The Intensive Care Unit is often a place of "intense" stress for the patient, the family members and the physicians. My office was on the same floor as the ICU, just outside the family waiting room. I saw day after, day, family members faced with uncertain conditions for their loved ones. Sometimes it was an unexpected accident that had left family members asking the age old question of "why", while other conditions were brought on by our body's state of deterioration. Many tears were shed in the hallway outside of my office.

The one thing I know about being in the ICU is that life still goes on all around you. My interaction with some of the patients or family members may have been very brief, maybe a smile, or a tissue, or a kind word, while others would walk into my office and pour out their heart about what was going on in their life. They all seemed to start their conversation the same way…"I don't know if you can help me…..". It seems that the ICU is a place where people need help and they need hope. Life experiences help shape who we are and I would like to think that this book is offering some encouragement and hope when you need it most.

You need to understand that you can make a difference in your health, but a greater lesson to be learned comes from understanding that God is also in control. Our hope and peace that comes during very difficult situations, has got to come from above. I have personally had experience with family members being in the ICU, and can tell you that the hours that you sit and wait, seem like days, and the weeks seem like months. Everything seems to be in the "wait and see" mode. Patients can make dramatic improvements in the ICU or turn the other way in an instant.

I knew a family that had received the call that their Mother had collapsed while at the hospital, and was now in the ICU. Family members came rushing to her bedside, for there is something inside of all of us that says "this is serious" when we get that kind of call. Although I knew this family, I could see their concern and love for their Mother as they gathered around her bedside. Their love was not new, but there was a sense of imminence as their Mother laid in the hospital bed. She was critical, by hospital standards, and unresponsive. Even though they could see what was going on, there were still many questions. It often comes down to the patient or family members being educated on the patient's condition and the treatment plan, but remember the 3rd leg of the medical plan is the support system. Especially in times like these, you need to have your support system close by, all the time.

Almost all of the people that walked through my office door needed questions answered. Some questions were very simple while others were very complex. It has been said that "the more we know about a topic, the less there is to be afraid of". Being informed does not totally take away the stress of being in the ICU, but it can help. Effective communication between the patient, family members, nurses and physicians is a very important part of the healing process for the patient and the family.

In some situations, the patient is unable to communicate, so family members must step in. Even when someone is in the hospital and can communicate, it is important for family members to be present most of the time. It is also helpful if you have a large family, that one person be willing to be the "contact" person for communication.

THE ICU AND YOUR MEDICAL PLAN

I once had a patient that had a husband, seven children (who all had spouses and children), and I could have spent most of my day talking to them, as they all came at different times and all wanted questions answered. I was able to still communicate with them, but helped them organize the information so everyone was on the same page. I have had many patients and family members thank me for the care I provided, but it was the family of the patient with seven children that actually came back to the hospital after their mother had past away and thanked me for the care I had provided. Their kind gestures reminded me why I do what I do.

ICU Organized

One thing that will help you and your support group stay organized in the ICU is to write everything down, in one central notebook, so the information can be shared with other family members and will give the nurse more time with the patient. Here are some general suggestions for family members and patients in the ICU:

- Have someone present most of the time if possible.
- Write everything down: Questions when you think of them, answers when you get them, who provided the answers and when.
- Document treatments : Medications, bandage changes, etc.
- Document if the patient's condition changes and what intervention was initiated related to this change.
- Document all tests, lab work and procedures that are done, along with the results.
- Obtain updates on the patient's condition while you were gone.
- Go over treatment plans with the physician.
- Designate a "contact" family member for large families.
- Take shifts if family members are available to keep your strength up.
- Document any confirmed infections that the family or visitors

should be aware of, and what precautions need to be taken.
- If you have a compromised immune system, avoid visiting the ICU unless necessary.
- Bring all legal documents with you to the hospital and provide them to the nurse at the time of admission. Power of attorney documents can be taken to the hospital anytime as they can be kept on file.

Understand that most ICU nurses and doctors have a wealth of experience and understanding, and have gone through additional training on how to take care of critical patients. The decision to place patients in the ICU is not made without appropriate considerations of the patient and the hospital resources. There are approximately 50,000 ICU beds across the United States, including specialty units like Cardiovascular ICU, Neonatal ICU, Neurological ICU and Surgical ICU. Most hospitals have a relatively small number of ICU beds in comparison to the rest of the hospital and the rooms are generally reserved for those who are most in need. After discussion about all the infectious diseases we could be exposed to in the hospital, the place carrying the highest risks to any patient is the ICU. It is true that patients in the ICU most likely have the highest physical impairment or system compromise of all patients. The question remains, is it the place or the patient that causes the highest risk for these nosocomial infections? The answer may be both. We do know that the ICUs that have implemented infection control measures have seen a decrease in their infection rate, but the patient's ability to fight off disease can also play a part.

Hospitals have different protocols for ICU requirements, but some of the scenarios that could place the patient in the ICU would be if they are:

- Intubated (needs assistance breathing)
- Receiving medications that are regulating their heart
- If they have a pulmonary artery line

THE ICU AND YOUR MEDICAL PLAN

- If they are 80 years old with heart or vascular conditions
- Surgical complications that require another surgery
- Continuous or ongoing bleeding
- Altered mental status chances
- After an organ transplant surgery
- Multiple trauma injuries

Hospitals can set up their own criteria for admission requirements, so what may put a patient in the ICU in one hospital, may not at another. No matter what bed you or your family member is admitted to in the hospital, communication remains one of the key components.

Ask questions and if you do not get them answered, ask someone else. The ICU patients are often facing life or death situations. If you are not happy with your care or progress, ask for a second opinion, and notify the unit manager or the patient advocate from the hospital regarding your concerns. It is possible that the lack of progress in your condition may be a result of malpractice, and could be changed if different treatments are initiated, so it does not hurt to ask.

Patients may also be limited to the number of visitors allowed at one time in the ICU. Items such as flowers and food are usually prohibited, so ask before bringing them in. Some hospitals provide areas for family members to stay the night, but not all. I know many family members that have slept on the chairs in the waiting room to be close to their family member. This is not the best scenario for anyone's health, so make sure to get the proper rest. The support system should provide the nurses with contact phone numbers if they are leaving the unit and let the nurse know to call if anything changes. If family members do not give the nurse permission to wake them in the middle of the night...they might not. Communicate what the expectations are for all of the staff and support system, to maintain an effective team.

Advanced Directives

Making medical decisions about your care could be one of the

◄ SURVIVING YOUR MEDICAL CRISIS

most important decisions you will ever make, but who will make those decisions if you are unable? One part of your support team is to surround yourself with people that have your best interest in mind, and this does not change when you are unable to make decisions. You need to plan for the day that you might lay unconscious in the hospital bed and the medical team is asking what they should do.

Families have been torn apart over this very situation if the patient has not provided their thoughts and wishes in writing ahead of time. I once took care of a patient that had been diagnosed with cancer that was not responding to the treatments, and had developed pneumonia. This was a life threatening situation as the patient was now unconscious, and decisions needed to be made. There were three children; one who was a physician, and very much aware of their Mother's status, and two others that were very emotionally attached to their Mother. The attending physician felt that the patient was not going to survive this situation, and recommended that the family speak with Hospice about end-of-life care.

The children all met with the Hospice physician and nurse and the decision was made, reluctantly, to put their Mother in Hospice care. A few hours after this decision was made, the patient was moving a little in bed, and the one daughter saw this as signs of improvement. She immediately responded with, "We need to get her out of Hospice, she is improving". The other children did not concur, and the battle began. You see, the Mother had no Advanced Directives or Medical Power of Attorney, to guide their decisions. In situations like this, it can be very stressful for everyone, but if you have the legal paperwork completed, it can reduce some of that stress. There are different legal documents that everyone should have completed as part of their medical portfolio.

Medical Power of Attorney

This legal document allows you to give permission for someone else to make healthcare decisions for you in the event that you are unable to make them for yourself. The individual that you select will only make healthcare related decisions granted by this document.

When selecting someone for this task, you should have someone that understands how you feel about your health and what your wishes are in quality-of-life situations. It is important to select someone that is able to make medical decisions based on your view point, and will be able to set their own views aside. This can be a difficult task for many family members, as they tend to have their own opinions on how or what should be done for their loved one. You can limit their decision making power or give them total control over your care; it is all up to you. It is even possible for you to specifically say that your representative will not have control over one certain decision.

Most patients have selected a spouse or family member for this position, but others have selected outside sources, such as attorneys or friends. The healthcare providers that are also taking care of you cannot be your legal appointee for your medical decisions. It is always a good idea when drafting this document that you also have someone as a back-up person, incase your first selection is unavailable.

The Living Will

This is a different document than your Medical Power of Attorney. The Living Will contains information on how you want to be treated when there appears to be no hope for a recovery. This document will answer questions like: Do you want to be kept alive by machines? Do you want to be revived if you are found without a pulse or respirations? You have control over what happens, even though you are not able to make these decisions at the time.

It is not necessary for you to involve an attorney, but they could provide all of these documents, and would direct you for a fee. Many of these standard forms can be located on the internet free of charge. Here are a few examples:

http://www.st-joseph.org/will/med_pr_attorney.pdf
http://www.findlegalforms.com/forms/advance-health-directive/
http://www.wvlegalservices.org/medpoa.pdf

A witness will need to be present at the time of the patient signing this document, but it cannot be a spouse, relative or the appointee. Check with the individual state to see if your legal documents are binding in that state. Discuss your decisions with your physician, and make sure that he understands your wishes. If there is a discord between you and your physician regarding these documents, you need to seek another physician that will respect your wishes.

Difficult ICU Decisions

Many patients may not come out of the ICU, and the family will need to make some difficult decisions if no Living Will or Power of Attorney documents have been drafted. If the patient is basically "alive" because of the machines, the family may be faced with the decision of "turning the machines off", which will usually end the patient's life. This can be a very difficult decision to make, and should only be made when all treatment options have been exhausted and test have been run. Second opinions can be utilized in these cases as well. The support group will need to gather the information, analyze it, and make an informed decision, but they should never feel rushed into making this decision.

If the patient does die while at the hospital for whatever reason, the family is usually given a short time to be with the patient, but the patient's body will need to be transported to the morgue within a reasonable amount of time. Most hospitals will respect that family could be on their way to the hospital, but they cannot leave the body in the room for the relatives that are traveling a distance.

Spending time with your deceased loved one, may provide closure, but remain conscious about any infectious disease that might still be on the patient. Just because the patient is gone, does not mean that all the bacteria has left.

Most hospitals participate in some organ donation program and if the patient is a candidate, the family may be contacted by a representative. The family has the right to refuse this, but the patient's wishes should be honored. Organ donation saves countless lives all the time, and your loved ones should know how you feel about this program ahead of time. This should also be discussed with your Medical Power of Attorney representative and family members.

The family or legal representatives will need to contact the funeral home, and then the funeral home will make arrangements with the hospital to pick up the patient's body. Many people pre-plan their funeral and have all the arrangements made prior to their death, which is very helpful to the family. If this is the case, the family members should be provided this information at the time the arrangements are made.

The patient's belongings need to leave the hospital with a family member or patient representative. The designated person will need to sign the release of personal belongings documentation, which states what items were provided to them at the time of discharge. Do not leave "Grandma's ring" on her finger, or anything else of value, as you never know who may come in contact with her body. You can always put the ring back on at the funeral home if you would like for her to be buried in it. Items of any value should never be at the hospital to begin with, and should be taken home at the time of admission if brought accidently.

CHAPTER 7

Preventative Treatments

There are certain risks associated with anyone being in the hospital that are not based on their exposure to bacteria. These conditions have been studied over the years and protocols have been developed to prevent them. Everyone needs to understand what these conditions are, what is being done to prevent them, and if the treatment is right for them.

Deep Vein Thrombosis (DVT) is often referred to as the "Silent Killer" that knows no age limit. David Bloom was an active 39 year reporter that was traveling to Iraq to cover a news story. After the long airplane ride, he had complained of pain behind his knee. He had spoke with physicians back here in the states, but David put his work ahead of his care and died, just like 200,000 other Americans with DVT complications will this year, according to the American Heart Association. It is estimated that 600,000 patients will develop a venous thromboembolism this year even with all the preventative measures many physicians are utilizing today.

Dr. Samuel Z. Goldhaber, an associate professor at Harvard believes that this is a "public health crisis" as some physicians have different opinions on which preventative treatments should be utilized even though the research evidence is direct about the methods that are most effective for preventing DVT formation. Some do not use any preventative measures, while others only use compression stockings or aspirin. Recommended protocols need to be adjusted for each patient's condition, but also remembering that these recommendations are based on best practice studies. This difference in opinion among physicians could also put the patient at a higher risk for developing a DVT. It is important to find out what drugs your physician uses to prevent DVT formation, along with the possible side effects prior to administration.

A DVT is a condition where a blood clot develops in one or more veins in your legs, arms, pelvis, neck or chest. These clots can cause damage to the vein, but can also "break away" from the development site and lodge in other organs, which can be life threatening. DVT occurs when blood "pools" and a clot develops. It can be caused from many conditions, but if the patient is on bedrest or is unable to move because of previous surgery or trauma, the risk for this condition goes up. Patients with congestive heart failure, cancer, obesity, pregnancy, nephrotic syndrome, estrogen use or those unable to walk, are also at greater risk. I had a patient once that had been on an anti-estrogen drug that developed DVT as a side effect of the drug. This was a life or death situation for her and if she had not come to the hospital when she did, the result could have been much different. Because of the wide assortment of causes for DVT, it is important to know the symptoms.

Symptoms

The patients often report a pain or dull ache in the affected limb, along with possible redness or swelling of the affected area. The calf or thigh is the most common place of development. There can be a partial or a complete blockage of the vein, so the symptoms can be very vague, or they are masked by the patient's condition. If there has been trauma to the affected area, it may already be painful, red and swollen. It is estimated that as many as half of all DVT cases do not have any symptoms, but the risk for complications still exist. If the clot travels to the lungs, and blocks a pulmonary artery or one of its branches, it is now called a Pulmonary Embolism (PE).

With a PE, the patient may develop sharp chest pain, shortness of breath, sweating, anxiety, coughing (which may contain blood), lightheadedness or loss of consciousness. There is also the possibility that the patient may not have any symptoms at all. Although less common, DVT blood clots can travel to the kidneys, heart or brain. If the clot lodges in the heart, the patient can experience a heart attack, and if it is in the brain, the result could be a stroke. Both of these cases also carry a high mortality rate. If the DVT is caught and treatment is initiated in a timely fashion, there is less than 1% chance of a PE developing, so diagnosis and treatment are very important.

Diagnosis

A **Duplex Ultrasound** is a painless test that shows images of the blood vessels and how well the blood is or is not flowing through the vessels. A radiologist will place gel on the patient's skin and then will glide the ultrasound around the suspected area to obtain "pictures" for analysis. This procedure is very safe and does not emit any radiation. Depending on availability, this can even be done in the physician's office.

It is sometimes necessary for a **Venography** to be performed, which allows the physician to view the possible blockage through an X-ray that is taken after a radioactive dye is injected into the patient's body. This test is very accurate, but can put the patient at risk for additional clot formations and exposes them to X-ray radiation.

Magnetic Resonance Imaging (MRI) can also be used to view detailed images in the body. It may be necessary for an injection which will allow more details of the vessels to be viewed. This test can be very expensive and is often used as a last resort, but it is very effective for DVT diagnosis.

Blood test can also show an abnormal level of the clot-dissolving substances called D dimer. Other conditions can cause this abnormal result so the test does not always indicate a DVT, but could be used as a screening tool for those at risk.

Complications

Pulmonary Embolism is the primary concern associated with DVT. Another condition called post-thrombotic syndrome can develop after a patient has had a DVT, causing leg swelling, pain and discoloration of the skin. In this condition, the DVT has caused damage to the vein and the blood flow in that area has been restricted. It may even take years for this condition to develop after the DVT has been diagnosed.

Treatment for DVT

The primary objective for DVT treatment is to stop the clot that the patient has from getting any larger or from developing into a PE. The usual regiment includes medications that cause the blood to "thin", which decreases the blood's ability to clot. Most patients with a DVT are started on Heparin either intravenously or by injection, followed by Coumadin which is taken orally. Blood samples will be collected to monitor the patient's clotting time and the medication may be adjusted to certain parameters for each patient's condition. It is possible that the patient could be on this medication for months. The physician may also want the patient to wear compression stocking to help with the circulation in their legs, which is considered a non-invasive treatment.

Invasive treatments may be necessary. Intravenous medications, which have a dissolving affect, may be injected close to the clot in severe cases. The serious side effects of these drugs usually limit this treatment to only patients with life-threatening conditions. A balloon angioplasty is a common procedure for a DVT in the iliac vein, but is generally not used for other areas. A filter can also be placed in the vena cave in the abdomen to "catch" any breakaway clots and prevent them from going to the patient's lungs. A surgical procedure to remove the clot may also be necessary for patients that cannot take the clot-dissolving drugs. No matter what the course of treatment entails, anyone with a DVT needs to ask questions.

It is very important to understand the risks associated with each of these treatments along with the benefits. Patient's with DVTs or those scheduled for surgery need to ask their physician what treatment will be utilized, the rationale behind the selection, what the risks are and how long the treatment will last. Some of the anti-coagulant medications have been associated with some serious side effects and patient deaths, so make informed decisions.

Prevention

Many surgeons will prescribe an anti-coagulant after surgery to prevent DVT formation. If you are taking these medications after surgery, make sure your blood is being monitored to maintain therapeutic levels as clots can form even if you are taking them. Vitamin K, which can be found in green leafy vegetables, can work against your anti-coagulant medications, so watch your intake.

It is also possible that your clotting time is too high and this puts you at risk if you are injured. I had a patient once that fell while on Coumadin and injured her hip. Because of a prolonged bleeding time, what would have been a "normal" bruise on her hip now covered a very large area from her hip to below her knee.

If you have had surgery or are sitting in one place for long periods of time, move your lower calf muscles and feet, as this helps to keep the blood circulating, and reduces the chances for clot formation. Get up and walk around as soon as possible after surgery to reduce DVT risk and the compression stockings should be applied before surgery if possible or soon thereafter. If you quit smoking, control your blood pressure and maintain a proper weight, your DVT risk will be also be reduced.

When traveling long distances make sure to walk around when you can or do lower extremity exercises. Avoid crossing your legs or socks that compress the circulation, and make sure you are adequately hydrated as dehydration causes the blood to thicken. Wear compression stockings as a preventative measure for long trips. Natural supplements like Garlic can also have a "blood thinning" effect, so let your doctor know if you are taking this supplement as it could interfere with your medications or decrease your body's ability to stop bleeding.

SURVIVING YOUR MEDICAL CRISIS

DVT considerations:
1. Know the signs and symptoms of a DVT and PE.
2. Seek immediate medical attention if symptoms develop.
3. Find out what treatment your physician prescribes to prevent a DVT from developing while you are in the hospital.
4. Take your anti-coagulant medication as prescribed as the dose could change daily.
5. Blood needs to be drawn regularly to make sure the clotting times are in a therapeutic range.
6. Understand the side effects of the anticoagulant medications.
7. Know the conditions or medications that put you at risk for DVT development.
8. If a surgical procedure is required because of a DVT, understand all of the possible complications.
9. Monitor your intake of green leafy vegetables if you are taking Coumadin, as vitamin K can reduce its effectiveness.
10. Quit smoking, maintain proper weight and control your blood pressure to reduce your risk.
11. Lower extremity exercises can keep the blood circulating during long travel periods or times of bedrest.
12. Avoid tight socks or clothing that compresses blood circulation.

CHAPTER 8

Emergency Room Strategies

Each year millions of Americans utilize Emergency Room (ER) services. Hospital shows on television have provided an often unrealistic picture of how the emergency room actually works. We could only wish that our condition could be fixed within an hour, like the TV shows. If you have ever been to an ER, it is anything but glamorous. The last time we needed to go the ER was for our daughter as she had taken an elbow to the nose in the 1st quarter of a girl's basketball game.

After the game it was evident that her nose was broke, and she complained of a severe headache, so off to the ER we went. I called a couple of the local hospitals and asked how busy their ER was. I know that can change in a minute, but the one hospital responded with, "we are swamped", while the other one said they were "just steady". It was not rocket science as to which one we would go to. It took a couple of hours even at the hospital that was not too busy for an X-ray and to see the physician. If you have the time to call and have a selection of facilities to choose from, it is not a bad idea to inquire prior to the visit, as it could save some time.

Many factors could bring someone to the ER, but some may not truly be an emergency situation. Many calls come into 911 operators each year for ailments that do not require emergency care. One of the most ridiculous calls that I have heard going to 911 was placed by a lady that said she did not get her chicken nuggets that she had ordered. This was an example of poor usage for our 911 system.

Many people may require medical care, but not emergency medical care. The ER physicians are often overwhelmed, with a long list of sick and agitated patients that are tired of waiting. The ER is not a place where only people with emergencies go, as patients with limited resources may also show up at the ER. If the patient has no insurance or physician to see, or no one else to call to take them for medical care, they will often end up in an ambulance at the ER. Because of this, the ER physicians see such a wide range of patients each day, and must be able to "treat" them all. On any given day, the average ER can see patients with sports injuries, burns, uncontrolled bleeding, difficult breathing, heart attacks, strokes, confusion, overdoses, food poisoning, fevers, sinus infections, allergic reactions, broken bones and those from car accidents, just to name a few.

Prioritizing all the patient conditions that walk through the ER doors is an analytical process. The hospital physician does NOT see patients in the order in which they arrived. The patient is assessed, evaluated, and prioritized. Initial assessments allow for each patient to be put into a category related to the level of care they need as listed below:

- Immediately life threatening
- Urgent, but not immediately life threatening
- Less urgent

This provides a generalized idea of what most facilities use for a priority analysis. Hospitals are able to provide different levels of care, so the hospital you are taken to in an emergency may or may not be able handle your emergency situation.

Level I Trauma Centers

Hospitals are rated by the different levels of trauma based on certain criteria like who is staffing the ER and what equipment they have at the facility to handle trauma cases. A Level I trauma center provides the highest level of surgical care and has a required number of physicians and anesthesiologist on duty at all times. Along with these physicians, prompt availability of specialty physicians can also be provided. Level I trauma centers will be more likely to have highly sophisticated medical diagnostic equipment, as it is more than just the average ER.

Each state can designate certain hospitals as trauma centers because they meet and follow the American College of Surgeon's recommendations for accreditation. Some hospitals are able to provide services that others are not qualified to provided. Our daughter's friend, John was involved in a serious head-on car accident. A physician from a Level I trauma center was a few cars behind the accident and rushed to John's aid. He immediately requested a life-flight helicopter which was able to transfer John for life saving treatments. John had sustained a spinal cord injury, and studies have shown good outcomes with early steroid treatment if provided within the first few hours after the accident. Had he been transferred to the local hospital by ambulance, and then transferred again to the Level I trauma center, that precious time could have been gone.

Level II

Level II hospitals usually work closely with a Level I center and can provide extensive trauma care. Essential specialties and equipment are available, but are not required to have any surgical residency or research program at the hospital.

Level III

This level hospital does not have the full availability of specialists, but can provide surgical procedures, resuscitation and intensive care for most patients. These facilities usually have some sort of agreement with a Level I or II facility for the ability to transfer critical patient once stabilized.

Level IV
This trauma center basically evaluated, stabilizes, utilizes diagnostic capabilities and then will transfer the patient to a higher level of care. It can provide necessary surgery or critical care to stabilize the patient. Trauma nurses and physician are usually available upon the patient's arrival, but the center also has an agreement with a higher level trauma center for patient transfers.

It is important to know what level of care your local hospital provides incase you ever need their services. We live in a metropolitan area where access to at least 10+ different hospitals is within 30 minutes from our home. Level I trauma centers offer more "services", but it does not always mean that your local facility cannot meet your needs. If the patient's condition is critical and could need immediate surgical interventions, the Level I may be the best bet if it is close by. Gathering information ahead of time will allow you to be prepared when that emergency situation occurs.

It is not a question of "if" you or one of your family members will need emergency services; it is a question of when. My parents had four children that grew up on a Quarter Horse farm in Ohio where we had mini-bikes, tractors, horses, dogs, cats and ATV's, but very few of these "high risk" activities took us to the hospital. Over a 40 year period, we have required ER services 17 times. I fell off my pony, which took a small step to one side, and I received six stitches in my chin. Yet, when a car pulled out in front of me when I was driving 65 miles an hour (before seat belt laws), I injured my knee, but did not require ER services. Go figure.

One of our most memorable ER visit was with my brother Chris. He was working for a construction company one summer building decks. He had his steel toed boots on, but somehow he touched the end of the electric nail gun to his foot as he reached for another board, and the gun fired a nail, and nailed his foot to the deck. The EMS and his co-workers cut the bottom of the board off the

EMERGENCY ROOM STRATEGIES

deck and took him to the ER, wood and all. A surgeon was called in as they tried to figure out how to remove the nail from his foot, boot and deck board. Because the steel toed boots also had a steel reinforcement in the bottom of the boot, they could not get an accurate X-ray, so the physician had to make a judgment based on his assessment. He didn't think the nail had hit any bones, but they would need to remove the nail to make sure. They just weren't sure what tool to use to remove the nail. My Uncle had a pair of pliers in his truck that the doctor eventually used to remove the nail. I am not sure if the physician did not have the right tools, but they got the nail out. This was not a life threatening situation and most local hospitals should have been able to handle this type of situation.

A friend of our family was working with his table saw when he accidently severed his hand. The community hospital that my brother went to was also the one our friend was taken to. They ended up transferring him by life-flight to a larger hospital for treatment. It just depends on each patient's condition and what the hospital is able to handle. If you are transported by ambulance, you may or may not have a say in which hospital they take you to, but researching the hospitals ahead of time could provide direction if that is a possibility. Visiting an ER can be stressful and traumatic so let's cover how the ER works and hopefully reduce some of the anxiety.

When to go to the ER

First of all, you need to decide if you actually need emergency care. Contacting your physician first for minor symptoms or questions could save you a lot of time and money. If you do not have a physician, there are walk-in clinics generally available in most cities. Some insurance companies provide a telephone nurse to answer your personal questions, so check with your provider to see if they offer this service. Some ERs have a specialty service for pediatrics, but may require you to be transferred to a pediatric hospital once stabilized. Many hospitals today offer observation units, where a patient's condition will be monitored and if it improves, will most likely be discharged. If the patient's condition does not improve, they may be admitted or transferred to another facility. Hospitals today are trying to deal with the influx of patients that are visiting the ER with less severe problems and may offer patients the "fast track" pathway. Realize that even though you are offered this, it does not guarantee that your visit will be "fast". If a trauma arrives, that situation can take staff from the "fast track" area to assist.

To assist the physicians, it is recommended that all individuals carry an "emergency folder", which includes a list of all your medications, supplements, insurance cards, names of your primary care physician, a list of any chronic conditions, surgical history and drug allergies. It is helpful if you frequent the hospital that you try and visit the same facility as they have access to all of your previous medical history, including labs and diagnostic testing. Having these resources can often reduce not only your time, but also the cost of your visit.

Staffing for the ER can also vary from hospital to hospital. Some hospitals may provide board certified ER physicians while others are regular hospital physicians that cover the ER on a rotation basis. Check with your local facility for staffing procedures if this is of concern to you. It is also possible that an agency nurse will be staffing the ER, but it does not mean that they have less knowledge, but they might not be as familiar with where things are at that hospital.

Course of Action

After the nurse has finished her initial assessment, the ER physician will collect more information and then formulates a list of possible causes of the patient's condition. If a diagnosis cannot be provided with just an exam, diagnostic test may be required. Hopefully the facility has the necessary equipment to perform the required test. At this point, if they do not have say the "MRI", the patient may be sent to another facility. Being aware of what equipment your local hospital has available ahead of time can prevent this scenario from occurring.

Even if they have the necessary equipment, it may take time for tests or lab work to be performed and evaluated, so plan on spending some time waiting. Bring a book or something to do while passing the time. Do not be afraid to ask about your insurance coverage before the tests are performed, as even though the hospital participates with your insurance, the physicians, or radiologist that are interpreting the test may not. These are good questions to ask before the tests are performed as there may be a less expensive alternative. There should also be social workers in the ER that can assist you with any insurance issues.

Once the patient has been treated and/or diagnosed, they will be discharged, admitted or transferred. If they are discharged, it may take a little while to receive all the necessary instructions and paperwork as the nurses and physicians are trying to take care of multiple patients. Before the patient leaves the hospital, make sure to fully understand any discharge instructions, have the names of all physicians that evaluated the case and understand all prescriptions that have been provided.

If you are being admitted, realize that this too may take a while before a bed is ready. Patients often arrive on the units after spending an extended amount of time in the ER, and those in observation could have been there for two to three days. Waiting for "something" to happen at the hospital is very common, but if you are hungry while waiting for a bed, make sure to ask your nurse or physician if you can have something to eat. If testing is still being performed, then it might not be possible for the patient to consume food. Many cafeterias are only open certain hours and if you arrive "after hours", you may only find the sandwich Dietary left in the unit's refrigerator. Be proactive in your care as the healthcare team may not have the same priorities that you have, or just are not thinking about you being hungry.

Results

Some studies have shown that just because you are taken to a Level 1 trauma center does not mean that you will be provided the "best" care. There are differences from one hospital to another, just like any other care, so the focus needs to be on the outcomes and not just on the number of physicians they have on hand.

I knew a patient that had visited the ER three times before she was diagnosed with a ruptured appendix. She was pregnant and had been sent home with antacids to treat the "pain" she was reporting. The lack of a correct diagnosis on the previous visits resulted in weeks in the hospital and a threat of antibiotics that could harm the baby. Remember that ER physicians see a lot of patients each day and can also make mistakes. If you have a condition that does not improve, gets worse, or you develop other symptoms, you need to be reevaluated.

Although the emergency medical services can be over-used, do not hesitate to call 911. I have always told my patients that chest pain, shortness of breath, moderate blood loss, loss of consciousness or trauma could all indicate that an ambulance is necessary, over someone driving you to the hospital. The patient becomes priority #1 when they arrive in the ambulance and the EMS workers can also provide life-saving treatments on the way to the hospital. The EMS workers are trained for these types of situations so if there is a question to call or not to call 911- CALL. It is better to be on the safe side than to have the physician say…."if you had only received medical treatment sooner…"

Considerations for Your ER Visit:
1. Plan ahead- Ask your physician which hospital he would recommend or that he has privileges at.
2. Carry with you an "Emergency Folder" filled with insurance information, medication list, physician's names and numbers, along with your medical and surgical history.
3. Locate the Level I trauma centers in your area, and find out what your local hospital is rated.
4. Patients are treated on a priority basis after a brief evaluation, so be patient if you are not critical.
5. Make sure to tell someone if your symptoms get worse or new ones develop while waiting to see a physician.
6. "Bugs" are in the ER too, so make sure your care providers wash their hands.

7. You and your visitors also need to have good hand hygiene to prevent infections.
8. Inquire about the status of the local hospital, ER physicians and radiologist participation with your insurance.
9. Ask if the ER physicians are board certified in ER medicine.
10. Call your physician or go to urgent care facilities for minor conditions.
11. If you are sick or injured, have someone take you to the hospital, or call 911 for emergency situations.
12. Do not be afraid to ask questions about tests and treatments, and possible alternatives.
13. If the ER physician wants to call in a specialist, you can request the physicians you want. If you do not have anyone to request, you will get who the ER doctor consults or the physician that is on-call.
14. Be patient as tests can take a while.
15. Bring something to read or do while waiting.
16. Ask for food if you are hungry. You may not be able to have anything during initial testing, but it is ok to ask.
17. Observation units are interim units to monitor your condition.

Conclusion

I have a lot of healthcare providers to thank for the wonderful care they have provided my family over the last 40+ years. We have put our lives in the hands of Neurosurgeons, Oncologist, Hematologist, Orthopedic Surgeons, Plastic/Reconstruction Surgeons, Pediatricians, Neurologist, Gynecologist/Obstetricians, Radiologist, Anesthesiologist, General Surgeons, Cardiologist, General Practitioners, Dermatologist, Podiatrist, Nurses, Nursing Assistants and Physical Therapist...to name a few. Through research, we have been blessed with very talented care providers, but the case is not the same for many individuals.

I have written this book to assist with your development of a strong support system for your medical needs. Maintaining a healthily life style is a wonderful practice, but in its simplistic manor, it does not apply to many situations. To maintain our health, we often require a hospital or physician, so we must be prepared.

Today, hospitals are striving to gain our business in many different ways. Some will build new buildings, or put new tile on the floor, but most people want more than these amenities. Even though money does play a factor into their strategy, if the patient is not at the "top of the list", word gets around. It is called their "reputation", and with the availability of more information published today, the hospitals will be required to step up their game plan. The public wants to know more information about the hospital and what the statistics say. They also want to know what other patients have to say about their hospital stay. The public has become wise consumers, not only of their money, but of their health, and their life. They want the best care that they can receive and will travel great lengths to obtain this care.

The hospital is the 1st leg of your medical plan. You need a clear picture of what the hospital has to offer in equipment as well as the staff available for your care. The hospitals you select need to meet or exceed your standards of care. Insurance companies can have an impact on the hospital availability, if you want them to assist with your bill, but make your voice heard if they are not willing to pay for your treatments. The insurance company is employed by you or your employer, but some times they forget that, so effective communication with your insurance company can insure that you will receive the necessary treatments.

The hospital should be there to serve you, and though it may seem like all the insurance companies are concerned about is money, they are actually making some decisions that could be beneficial to the patient in the long run. By placing parameters related to pressure ulcers or hospital acquired infections, the insurance mandates, may actually force the hospitals to make more preventative measures part of their policies. If the insurance companies are not willing to pay for your treatment, then that too, could be a problem, because you may get stuck with the bill. The hospital should be willing to stand up for you as well as your insurance company, but no one will be concerned about your health like you will.

Some insurance companies do not directly regulate patient care, but they can make regulations that force the hospital to make cuts in the staff which ultimately affect the way you are cared for. Patient's acuity levels are on the rise, more documentation is required of the staff, and the number of patients a care provider is responsible for is going up. This scenario does not allow for patients to receive the best care possible. Be your own patient advocate and stand up for what you expect from your insurance company and your hospital.

The next leg of your healthcare plan consist of your physician and healthcare providers, as they have the most direct impact on the care you will receive during your medical crisis. Select someone that is willing to treat you as they would their dearest loved one. I have told many people that I look at my patients as though it were my Mother lying in that hospital bed. I love her more than I could express, and that has an impact on how I treat my patients. You should expect no less from your care providers.

There is a shortage of family practitioners or regular medical doctors, and many of those will be retiring soon. It may not be an easy task to locate a physician that will be your "health partner". He or she is the director, the manager or the controller of your health and ultimately, your life. This decision is a key element in developing a successful healthcare team. If you have not found that perfect physician, keep looking, as they are out there waiting for you to find them.

The third leg of your healthcare plan is the people that you surround yourself with; those friends and family members that truly care about your wellbeing. There are life-giving people and life-draining people, so make sure that you have the right ones around you. Appoint a Power of Attorney that will be able to make decisions related to your healthcare and document what your wishes are, to avoid any misinterpretation. Anyone in the middle of a medical crisis needs encouragement. Make sure to look for resources in your family, friends, church, support groups and from God.

The forth leg of the healthcare plan is YOU! We make decisions everyday, but many are not as important as our healthcare decisions. To be an effect part of your team, you must know about your health condition, the options for treatments and the risks associated with your care. We cannot sit back while others make decisions about our care, we must take an active part. Know your risks and how to prevent unwarranted things from happening to you. Physicians make decisions based on their experience and it is important that you feel comfortable with the decisions that they make. We need to be an active part of the healthcare team, ask questions and make informed decisions.

Millions of patients are treated every year, and many will not survive because they have not been prepared for their medical crisis. We need to take off the rose colored glasses and realize that it is not a matter of if we will need medical services, but the question is when. The ultimate healthcare plan consists of:

The Right Hospital
The Right Physicians and Healthcare Providers
(Doing the right things, at the right times)
The Right Support Group
And YOU!

Medical Plan Summary

1. Finding the right hospital will require some exploration along with analysis of the information to determine if the facility meets your standards of care.
    a. How many beds does the hospital have?
    b. Is the hospital a teaching facility?
    c. If it is a teaching hospital, what schools do they partner with?
    d. How many residents do they have at the hospital?
    e. What specialties (Surgery, OB/GYN, etc) have residents?
    f. What diagnostic equipment do they have on site?
    g. What types of Specialist are on staff 24/7?
    h. What is the hospital's infection rate?
    i. Does the hospital see enough patients to report for the CMS information?
    j. What areas does the hospital not meet the required reporting for the CMS?
    k. Are the results of the CMS and JCAHO reports positive?
    l. Did surgical patients receive antibiotics within 1 hour of their surgical incision?

    m. Did heart attack patients receive necessary treatments?
    n. Has there been any sentinel events at this hospital?
    o. Is the hospital JCACHO or AOA approved?
    p. What is the hospital's mortality rate on the CMS reports?
    q. What is the rating given to physicians and nurses from the patients?
    r. Do the patients find the rooms clean?
    s. Was the patient's pain controlled?
    t. What specialties have been recognized as a Center of Excellence?
    u. Does your physician have privileges to practice at this hospital?
    v. Are the rooms private or semi-private?
    w. Your thoughts after personally visiting the hospital?
    x. How many miles is this hospital from your home?
    y. Is the hospital participating in clinical studies?
    z. Does the hospital accept your insurance?

2. **Finding the right physician that meets your needs will require investigation of the physician along with a possible interview before establishing a relationship.**

    a. Is the physician a Medical Doctor (MD) or a Doctor of Osteopathy (DO)?
    b. Are they in a group or individual practice?
    c. Who covers for them when they are gone?
    d. What types of insurance do they accept?
    e. How long have they been practicing?
    f. What is their area of specialty?
    g. Where did they go to medical school and perform their residency?
    h. What are their office hours?
    i. Where are they located?
    j. What hospitals do they have privileges at?
    k. If you wanted an appointment, how soon would you be able to see them?
    l. Is it a male or female?
    m. What types of services do they offer in their office (x-ray, lab, etc)?

n. What awards or recognitions have they received?
o. What languages does the physician speak, and what is their primary language?
p. What ratings does the physician receive on HealthGrades or other websites?
q. How many patients do they see each day in their office?
r. What do other patients have to say about the physician?
s. Does the physician practice at a hospital that meets your standards of care?
t. Has the physician ever had any disciplinary actions taken against them?
u. Who recommends this physician?

Keep a list of the physicians you would like to take care of you in your medical portfolio.

Specialist	Physician's Name
General Surgeon	
Pulmonologist (Respiratory)	
Neurologist (Nerves/Brain issues)	
Orthopedic (Bones)	
Cardiologist (Heart-Circulatory)	
Hematologist/Oncologist (Blood-Cancer)	
Nephrologists/Urologist (Kidney)	
Pediatrics (Children/Babies)	

3. **Finding the right support group can provide peace of mind when you do experience a medical crisis. Planning for that day will reduce the stress associated with unplanned events.**

    a. Appoint a Medical Power of Attorney that will carry out your wishes when you are unable to make decision regarding your health. This will require you to fill out the necessary legal documents.
    b. Surround yourself with life-giving people that will have your best interest in mind.
    c. Select people for your support group that you can count on to be there during your medical crisis, for moral, physical and spiritual support.

4. **Become an educated patient on your diseases and conditions. You will then be able to be an active part of your medical team and make informed decisions regarding your health.**

    a. Develop a complete Medical Portfolio for your medical future.
    b. Information on diseases and medical conditions is available on the internet, libraries, and magazines, along with many community education centers.
    c. Know how to protect yourself and your loved ones from hospital acquired infections.
    d. Take a preventative approach to your health by exercising, eating the right foods and reducing your stress and you could save yourself from a medical crisis.

Terms to Know

AMI- Acute Myocardial Infarction or more commonly known as a heart attack. A coronary artery occlusion has occurred and blocks the blood flow to that area of the heart.

Abdomen- The area between your pelvis and your chest.

ABG- Arterial Blood Gas.

Adhesion- The band that holds parts together that may generally be separated.

Airway obstruction- Something that prevents air from flowing in and out of the airways.

Angina pectoris- A pain or pressure in the chest due to inadequate blood flow to the muscles of the heart.

Aneurysm- An abnormal weakening of a blood vessel.

Aspiration- Inhalation of food or liquids into the lungs.

Afebrile- The absence of fever.

Angiography- A test that shows the blood vessels by an X-ray. It can show possible blockages in the vessels.

Angioplasty- A surgical procedure in which a tube catheter is inserted into a section of your artery that has been narrowed due to

disease. A balloon will be inflated at the narrow point to open the artery.
Anticoagulent- Medication used to prevent blood clots.
Antiemetic- Medication used to treat nausea or vomiting.
Arrheythmias- Abnormal heart beats.
Atypical- Deviating from a normal state.
Arthrocentesis- Removal of fluid from a joint by a needle.
Ascites- Fluid collecting in the abdominal cavity.
Asepsis- Without infection
Barium- A chemical used to assist with X-ray diagnosis.
Benign- Not malignant- Non cancerous.
Biopsy- A procedure where a small amount of tissue is collected for examination under a microscope for evaluation of malignancy.
Bone Marrow- Soft tissue in the inside of the bones.
Bowel obstruction- A blockage in the intestines that prevents the moving of stool through the intestines in a proper manner.
Bronchoscopy- A procedure where a instrument is passed down the throat to study the air passages of the lungs.
Bypass- A procedure that allows fluid to flow past an obstructed area, which is done in a coronary artery bypass.
CABG- Coronary artery bypass graft.
Carcinoma- Cancerous or malignant growth.
Cardiac Cath- A procedure where a tube is inserted into a blood vessel and travels to the heart to evaluate its functionality.
CAT Scan- A diagnostic test that uses multiple X-ray pictures to produce slice-like views.
Catheter- A tube that is inserted into the body that can allow drainage, or injection of treatments.
CBC- Stands for Complete Blood Count. Common blood work performed for evaluation of a patient's condition.
Clinical Pathway- A printed guideline of usual care provided for

a patient having a certain procedure done or disease/condition.

Colonoscopy- A procedure that allows the physician to see inside of the intestines.

Coronary Arteriography- An Angiography of the heart muscle.

CPR- Cardiopulmonary resuscitation that is performed as part of an emergency response system.

Culture- When tissue or material is collected for examination under a microscope for microorganisms or living cells.

Cyanosis- Discoloration of the skin or lips, which results due to the lack of oxygen.

Diastolic- The lower number on your blood pressure.

Dysuria- Difficult or painful urination.

Echocardiography- Examination of the heart using ultrasound waves.

Embolism- A blood clot that has broken away from the orginal location.

EMR- Electronic Medical Record.

Endoscope- A procedure where a tube is inserted into the body and allows the physician to view or even take pictures of certain tissues.

Fibrillation- A rapid vibration or quivering of the heart muscle.

Graft verses host- Occurs when a transplant or transfusion is attacked by the recipients' body.

Hematoma- A swelling filled with blood in an organ or tissue

Hemorrhage- Excessive blood loss.

Holistic- Treatments that are believed to be of nature.

Intravenous Infusion- Commonly referred to an IV. Medications, vitamins, saline or other liquids are infused from a bag, into a vein.

Latent- To lay quiet, not active.

Lumbar puncture/Spinal tap- A needle is inserted between the vertebrae and a small amount of cerebrospinal fluid is abstracted for examination.

MRI- Magnetic Resonance Imaging. A device that scans the body using a magnetic field and radiofrequency.

Malignant- Cancerous

Nasograstric tube- A tube that is placed through the nose and into the stomach. It can be used for both draining purposes or for transferring food.

Mammogram- An X-ray of the breast used for cancer screening.

Needle biopsy- A small tissue sample extracted by a needle for examination.

Nosocomial infections- Infections that are acquired from the hospital setting.

NPO- Nothing by mouth.

Paracentesis- Removal of fluid from the body for therapeutic or diagnostic purposes.

Plasma- Component of the blood that carries water and nutrients to your tissues while its' proteins also help your blood to clot

Platelets – The "sticky" part of your blood with the main function being to stop bleeding.

Prophylactic- Treatment provided to prevent a disease or condition from occurring.

TPN- Total Parenteral Nutrition. Nutritional substances that are usually administered via an IV.

Red blood cells- The transporters of the oxygen to the tissue and organs, and also takes the carbon dioxide back to the lungs

Remission- A time where previous disease is not present.

Renal failure- The kidney's fail to function properly.

Sepsis- Infection or toxins have spread throughout the body.

Sputum- Mucus expelled from the lungs.

Stenosis- A narrowing of a vessel.

Stomach tube- A tube place through the abdominal wall and into the stomach generally used for feeding purposes.

Stress Test – A test used to measure cardiovascular fitness.

Syncope- Fainting or loss of consciousness.

Systolic- The top number of your blood pressure.

Tachycardia- Fast abnormal heart beats, generally over 100 beats per minute.

Thoracentesis- When fluid is abstracted from the chest.

Thrombus- A blood clot.

Transient Ischemic Attack- (TIA) Is consider a "mini stroke", that occurs when there is a blockage or spasm of an artery in your brain.

Ultra sound- A diagnostic test used to view internal tissue using cyclic sound pressure.

Upper GI study- A series of X-rays and fluoroscopic of the stomach, and duodenum after ingestion of a substance like barium.

White blood cells- Are responsible for protecting the body from infection and foreign material.

www.ingramcontent.com/pod-product-compliance
Lightning Source LLC
Chambersburg PA
CBHW071417170526
45165CB00001B/305